'An engaging and accessible book, which provides a "can do" perspective on the delivery of person-centred dementia care. This book provides practical examples and scenarios to help care providers think through best practice approaches to a range of everyday and more complex situations. As such it is a must-have book for anyone providing care for people living with dementia.'

— *Dr Claire Surr, Reader in Dementia Studies, Bradford Dementia Group, University of Bradford, UK*

'Our ultimate goal should always be to positively enrich and enhance the lives of people living with dementia. Caroline has made achieving this possible through this very practical and step-by-step guide to implementing a person-centered care approach. Based on her many years of hands-on experience and extensive work within the dementia care field, this is a "must have" for anyone rendering care. Highly recommended!'

— *Karen Borochowitz, Executive Director at the Dementia SA Team, South Africa*

Developing Excellent Care for People Living with Dementia in Care Homes

Bradford Dementia Group Good Practice Guides

Under the editorship of Professor Murna Downs, Chair in Dementia Studies at the University of Bradford, this series constitutes a set of accessible, jargon-free, evidence-based good practice guides for all those involved in the care of people with dementia and their families. The series draws together a range of evidence including the experience of people with dementia and their families, practice wisdom, and research and scholarship to promote quality of life and quality of care.

Bradford Dementia Group offer undergraduate and post-graduate degrees in dementia studies and short courses in person-centred care and Dementia Care Mapping, alongside study days in contemporary topics. Information about these can be found at www.bradford.ac.uk/health/dementia.

other books in the series

Leadership for Person-centred Dementia Care
Buz Loveday
Foreword by Professor Murna Downs
ISBN 978 1 849052 290
eISBN 978 0 857006 912

Risk Assessment and Management for Living Well with Dementia
Charlotte L. Clarke, Heather Wilkinson, John Keady and Catherine E. Gibb
Foreword by Professor Murna Downs
ISBN 978 1 849050 050
eISBN 978 0 857005 199

Person-centred Dementia Care
Making Services Better
Dawn Brooker
ISBN 978 1 843103 370
eISBN 978 1 846425 882

Enriched Care Planning for People with Dementia
A Good Practice Guide to Delivering Person-centred Care
Hazel May, Paul Edwards and Dawn Brooker
ISBN 978 1 843104 056
eISBN 978 1 846429 606

Involving Families in Care Homes
A Relationship-centred Approach to Dementia Care
Bob Woods, John Keady and Diane Seddon
ISBN 978 1 843102 298
eISBN 978 1 846426 780

Developing Excellent Care for People Living with Dementia in Care Homes

Caroline Baker

Foreword by Professor Murna Downs

Jessica Kingsley *Publishers*
London and Philadelphia

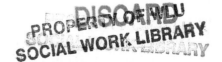

Figure 3.1 on page 58 is reproduced with permission from iStockphoto®.

First published in 2015
by Jessica Kingsley Publishers
73 Collier Street
London N1 9BE, UK
and
400 Market Street, Suite 400
Philadelphia, PA 19106, USA

www.jkp.com

Copyright © Caroline Baker 2015
Foreword copyright © Murna Downs 2015

Front cover image source: Thinkstock®. The cover image is for illustrative purposes only, and any person featuring is a model.

Library of Congress Cataloging in Publication Data
Baker, Caroline, 1964- author.
  Developing excellent care for people with dementia living in care homes / Caroline Baker.
    p. ; cm. -- (Bradford Dementia Group good practice guides)
  Includes bibliographical references and index.
  ISBN 978-1-84905-467-6 (alk. paper)
  I. Title. II. Series: Bradford Dementia Group good practice guides.
  [DNLM: 1. Dementia--nursing--Great Britain--Case Reports. 2. Homes for the Aged--standards--Great
Britain--Case Reports. 3. Aged--Great Britain. 4. Patient Care Planning--standards--Great Britain--Case
Reports. 5. Patient-Centered Care--methods--Great Britain--Case Reports. WT 27 FA1]
  HV1454.2.G7
  362.1968'3--dc23
                                2014020814

British Library Cataloguing in Publication Data
A CIP catalogue record for this book is available from the British Library

ISBN 978 1 84905 467 6
eISBN 978 1 78450 053 5

Printed and bound in Great Britain by Bell & Bain Ltd, Glasgow

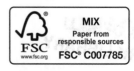

For Mum and Dad, Ian and Tara.

*In loving memory of my much missed
and much loved Grandparents.*

*None of this would be possible without any one
of you who have taught me that sharing good
things brings out the very best in people.*

*The proceeds from this book will be distributed between
St. Giles Hospice Lichfield and Dementia SA.*

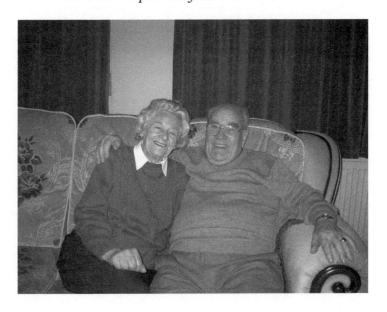

Contents

Foreword by Professor Murna Downs   9

Acknowledgements   11

Introduction   15

Chapter 1   Person-centred Care in Practice   21

Chapter 2   Nothing About Me Without Me   35

Chapter 3   Life Story and Lifestyle   49

Chapter 4   Person-centred Planning   61

Chapter 5   Getting the 'Fundamentals' Right   73
            Sue Goldsmith

Chapter 6   Making the Most of Mealtimes   89
            Jason Corrigan

Chapter 7   Reducing Distressed Reactions   105

Chapter 8   Reviewing the Use of Anti-psychotic
            Medication   119
            Dr Pete Calveley

Chapter 9   Developing the Environment: Providing
            a Supportive Environment   129

Chapter 10 Supporting Staff   147
            Jason Corrigan

Chapter 11 Proactive Analysis and Follow-through   161
            Sue Goldsmith

Chapter 12 Celebrating Success   181

            References   195

            Index   199

Foreword

It is now widely acknowledged that many of the most frail and vulnerable people with dementia live and die in care homes. Yet quality of life and quality of care in these settings continues to be an international concern. Poor care has been amplified time and time again by the media – whether in newspapers or on television. However well-intentioned these exposés may be, they do not in and of themselves help to provide good care, never mind excellent care. Indeed, an untoward side effect of these media portrayals is that care homes carry almost as much stigma as having dementia. We are in a position of a double whammy of low expectations – having dementia and living in a care home.

It is now timely to present a more optimistic yet achievable picture of the potential for living well in a care home. *Developing Excellent Care for People Living with Dementia in Care Homes* provides this alternative, optimistic view of living a good life until you die in a care home. It provides valuable practical guidance and suggestions for care home providers, staff and people affected by dementia. Informed by the theoretical underpinnings of person-centred care, the book not only describes person-centred care in practice but most importantly how it can be achieved and embedded into day-to-day practice.

We are familiar with the enthusiasm many feel for the person-centred approach. *Developing Excellent Care for People Living with Dementia in Care Homes* provides an overview of tried-and-tested strategies which have been used to achieve and embed sustainable change in practice. In this way, the initial motivation to provide person-centred care leads to sustainable change in practice. For too long we have expected care staff to be able to apply and embed person-centred care. We now recognise the need for organisational support and the need for the adequacy of such support to be audited.

Perhaps one of the most salient features of *Developing Excellent Care for People Living with Dementia in Care Homes* is that its author, Caroline Baker, is an acknowledged expert in the real world provision of person-centred care for people with dementia. She herself works for a large care home chain and has faced the kinds of challenges and seized the opportunities documented in this practice guide. It is timely that we hear from experts in the care home industry who not only recognise the value of a person-centred approach but who have worked over a period of many years to identify and embed strategies to realise its full potential for people with dementia and their families.

Professor Murna Downs
University of Bradford, August 2014

Acknowledgements

This book is a true consolidation of the knowledge and practice that I have developed over many years, none of which would have been possible without experts in their field who have guided me. The people below whom I would like to acknowledge have shaped my thinking in so many different ways – this book really would not have been possible without any one of them (and many whom I cannot mention without writing another book!).

First and foremost, my parents, Shirley and John Sewell, who have guided me, supported me and let me fly as free as a butterfly without admonishing any idea that I have come up with, but nurtured and praised and always demonstrated immense pride in everything I have done. You are (and will always be) my role models.

Second (and only because you came along later!), my husband Ian and my beautiful daughter Tara, who have also given me complete freedom in my career, realising that dementia care is my passion. You have supported me, praised me and never moaned when I am home very late or up in my office writing away at assignments, projects or books!

My dear brother, Tony Sewell – I was determined to go one better than your BSc Hons! I so admired your determination and success (and still do). Thank you for being my driving force. And Edel, my sister-in-law, thank you for proofreading some of my earlier chapters to let me know I was on the right lines, and for being so positive in your critique.

I began my nursing career at St Matthew's Hospital in Burntwood, where my passion for improving dementia care began, thanks to the inspirational lectures from the tutors at the nursing school and the role models I followed, in particular, my mum, Vanessa Scott, Kate Derry and Chris Beasley. And thank you to Diane Tongue, my study companion and true friend in nursing school.

Whilst working for the ExtraCare Charitable Trust, I was immensely inspired by John Graham, CEO of the organisation, who believed anything was possible and that we just had to work out how to make it happen. He agreed to fund my first big project as manager of a care home, a fully fitted-out sensory room costing an enormous amount of money. That taught me a big lesson, that actually, anything was possible if it was going to make a difference.

Within Walsall Primary Care Trust (PCT), John Farmer and Fiona McGill were champions of our projects and helped us to make them happen, which in turn, helped to improve the lives of hundreds of people living with dementia and their carers. I also had a fabulous team who shared the passion to get it right – Anne Shippey, Maria Whitehouse, Mandy Beck and Gail Lister.

Following a two-year secondment to Bradford Dementia Group, I am indebted to my colleagues who shared their vast knowledge of both person-centred care and evidence-based nursing practices – in particular, Paul Edwards, Dr Claire Surr, Professor Murna Downs and a special mention for Professor Dawn Brooker (now Director of the Association of Dementia Studies, Worcester University), who helped us to align the current criteria to her published work.

Last, but not least, I am incredibly proud to acknowledge the support and commitment of a number of people who have worked alongside me over the past nine years in Four Seasons Health Care to really make a lasting difference in dementia care: initially, Lou Smith, former Managing Director (MD) of the company who took me on and immediately listened to the need for further development and started us on our pathway. The Dementia Care Team was initialised with myself and Sharon Jones, who initially joined us a dementia care trainer, but also enthusiastically helped me to carry out the pilot of the PEARL (Positively Enriching And enhancing Residents' Lives) programme. Little did we know then that there would now be 70 validated homes, with another 70 on the programme! Julia Clinton, who became MD of the England division and a sincere champion of the PEARL programme – a true professional with a heart of gold. Dr Pete Calveley, our CEO, who supported, encouraged and educated us along our journey to define the programme we now have. I would also like to thank the current Senior Management Team for their support and guidance, especially Pauline Lawrance and Mike O'Reilly, who have provided direct line management, sound advice, encouragement and support over the past two years.

And last, but definitely not least, the outstanding Dementia Care Services Team, who are the most flexible, committed and passionate individuals I have worked with, and so rightly have won numerous awards.

A special mention for both Jason Corrigan and Sue Goldsmith (Heads of Dementia Care), who have both been 'my rock' for the past few years, and have overseen and helped the programme continue to develop. I am so glad that they have been able to be part of this publication.

A very special mention for Kate Marchant, my PA, without whom I would drown! For your humour, personality, enthusiasm, tenacity, flexibility and standard of work, I will forever be in your debt.

I would also like to thank Kate's husband, the late Tim Marchant (a former social worker) who read the initial chapters and provided such positive and detailed feedback. Your closing statement will always make me smile!

Introduction

It is estimated that over two-thirds of people currently living within care homes have a form of dementia, and of the 800,000 people with a diagnosis of dementia, one-third live within a care home (Alzheimer's Society 2012).

Moving into a care home can be a really difficult decision for some, and for relatives and friends of those who are caring for someone living with dementia. This can be especially difficult, as often the person being cared for may not be able to assist in the decision.

Most often, a person with dementia is admitted into a care home in the later stages of their illness, when the person who had been caring for them in a community setting is finding it more and more difficult to cope and is, perhaps, compromising their own health.

It is therefore incredibly important that the care home tries to replicate the person's own home as far as possible; gone are the days of institutional care and 'nameless faces'. Dementia care is no longer seen as the 'Cinderella' part of the health service, but a progressive, specialist field.

I currently work for Four Seasons Health Care, a large care home provider with over 450 homes across the UK; 250 of these provide dementia care. Over the past four years, we have developed the PEARL (Positively Enriching And enhancing Residents' Lives) programme that has enabled nearly 70 of these homes to become specialist dementia care units, with a further 70 currently going through the programme. The PEARL programme has won several awards and has been shortlisted for many others.

Many people suggested that I write this book so that as a company we can share the secrets of the programme that has seen many successes, including an average reduction of 50 per cent in the use of anti-psychotic medication as well as increases in residents' weight and well-being.

Most of the homes have taken 12 months to develop their units and truly embed the ethos of person-centred dementia care, and these homes have continued to develop their units, progressing to achieve even higher 'excellence' ratings. The homes work against 150 criteria, most of which are included within the text of this book and which were developed with Professor Dawn Brooker, utilising her VIPS framework approach (Brooker 2007) as our underpinning model.

There are many measurable successes within the programme, but some of the bigger successes are quite difficult to capture – dementia care units that are calm and relaxed, staff working alongside each other in a person-centred way, residents feeling as if they really are at home, relatives and friends feeling both included and involved.

AIM OF THIS BOOK

This book aims to highlight the key features of the programme, enabling staff within any care home to implement some of the interventions and practices that we have been able to demonstrate help to make a remarkable shift, from good fundamental care to specialist dementia care.

What we have realised over the past few years is that we can implement all of the ideas that can enhance quality of life, but without embedding the training in person-centred approaches and the understanding of how it may feel to be living with dementia, the 'softer touches', such as the environment and the range of activities, will not change the type of care that is given.

It is important that, after reading this book, each home develops their own criteria to align to their own ethos of care or mission statement, and that the criteria that they decide on will work on the ground with the resources they have.

Unfortunately, we have seen much in the media over the past few months of establishments that have unscrupulous staff within them. No excuses can be made for their behaviour, only real sadness that it happened at all. It is wholly understandable that those wishing to place their loved ones in a care home may have some serious reservations about entering one, but the places we see on the television are fortunately very few and far between. Most of us love and care deeply about we do, and our only ambition is to get it right.

People living with dementia are going to have a tough time at some point in their journey. Our job is to try to anticipate that fear or anxiety and to work alongside the person to help them feel safe or more confident, to help people retain their skills, to help them to live their life.

CONTENT

In Chapter 1, I provide an overview of how person-centred care can work in practice. Many care staff are sceptical, believing that person-centred care takes much more time and many more staff, but if we get it right, the opposite is true, since we work with the residents we are caring for rather than against them. The term 'person-centred care' has been coined in many mission statements and strategies, but we need to know what it actually means and how care can be transformed when we get it right.

In Chapter 2, I describe how we can try to involve the person living with dementia in the care home to help them to reach decisions about the care that they would like to receive. Gone, thankfully, are the days that we 'do for' and 'at' people living with dementia. Even for those residents who are in the advancing stages of their diagnosis, it is still possible to try and elicit their views of how they would like to receive their care through enhanced communication skills and specialist tools such as Dementia Care Mapping™ (DCM). This chapter also looks at the Mental Capacity Act 2005 and at how it can assist us in providing care for residents who may lack capacity.

In Chapter 3, I explore how our life story shapes the people we are, and how parts of our life story are critical to how we may want (or not want) to receive care. This chapter describes ways in which we might gather life story information and, equally as important, how we might transfer the knowledge into everyday care.

In Chapter 4, I consider the true meaning of a person-centred plan, and how it differs from a traditional care plan. This chapter has been written to help staff and relatives/friends to put together care plans with meaning, that are achievable and that will truly help the person living with dementia in the care home environment, using life story work.

In Chapter 5, Sue Goldsmith describes the importance of getting the 'fundamentals' of care right, and explains what the fundamental aspects of care are. If we are applying a person-centred approach, we need to take a holistic view of the person's needs in order to optimise their opportunity for well-being.

In Chapter 6, Jason Corrigan looks at the mealtime experience within the care home, and describes how we have implemented research and evidence-based practice to improve nutrition and, ultimately, helped our residents to gain weight. Most of us enjoy our meals and look forward to dining out in particular, and this should not be any different for a person living with dementia in a care home. Historically, it has been a given that people with a diagnosis of dementia will lose weight because of their condition. However, the elements that we have implemented within our programme have shown that a vast majority of residents will actually increase their weight. Jason describes how this may be achieved.

In Chapter 7, I explore whether most episodes of distress are avoidable, or at the very least, whether we might prevent episodes of distress becoming unmanageable, without the use of sedating medication. This chapter looks at how we can use non-pharmacological approaches that can help to reduce episodes of anxiety and distress. This is often referred to by many as 'challenging behaviour', but within the PEARL programme, we have purposefully lost this term to change the culture within the teams away from 'blame the resident' to almost self-blame. What did we miss?

In Chapter 8, Dr Pete Calveley looks primarily at how we might begin the process of anti-psychotic medication reduction within the care home. There has been a huge government drive to reduce the use of anti-psychotic medication for many reasons that will be explained within this chapter. In order to reduce its use, the programme has helped staff to look at alternatives, and to look at episodes of distress that may arise for other reasons. Too often in the past staff have turned to general practitioners (GPs) for 'sedating' medication to help them out of a crisis, whereas in fact, sometimes the medication itself can cause further distress.

In Chapter 9, I describe what we have found to be helpful (and what has worked) within the dementia care environment. There are lots of ideas within this chapter that have really helped to 'calm' the environment and help people to find their way around the care home. This chapter also looks at the types of activities that can be beneficial within the care home.

In Chapter 10, Jason Corrigan looks at how we can support staff to feel confident and capable to care for someone living with dementia. This chapter provides an introduction to the types of learning that have been helpful to us within our programme, such as the DCM, person-centred care, person-centred planning, resident experience training, supervision and post-incident support.

In Chapter 11, Sue Goldsmith provides an overview of how the care home should be monitoring their care, for example, reviewing the number of falls and distressed reactions, maintaining pain relief and weight, and what should be done if any adverse patterns are highlighted. This chapter also describes some of the specialist tools that might be used to provide proactive care that have not already been mentioned within the previous chapters.

In Chapter 12, in conclusion, I provide some insights from our residents, relatives and staff as to how the programme has made such a positive difference, and offer some thoughts as to how a care home might take the next steps to becoming a Centre of Excellence for People Living with Dementia.

Chapter 1

Person-centred Care in Practice

In this chapter, I provide an overview of how person-centred care can work in practice. Many care staff are sceptical, believing that person-centred care takes much more time and many more staff, but if we get it right, the opposite is true, since we work with the residents we are caring for rather than against them. The term 'person-centred care' has been coined in many mission statements and strategies, but we need to know what it actually means and how care can be transformed when we get it right.

The phrase 'person-centred care' often 'trips off the tongue' and is used within mission statements, government publications and advisory leaflets, seeming to have replaced 'individualised care' as a strapline. As a result, the many and varied interpretations of person-centred approaches can leave staff a little bewildered as to what it actually is and how to apply it to practice.

Throughout this book, I provide examples of how we implement person-centred care in practice. It is complex in as much as there are so many facets to ensure that we include everything and leave little to chance.

Person-centred care is the only way forward – there is no going back – and we have seen how rich the outcomes of this approach can be: residents who feel happy and well cared for and who are, as much as possible, able to manage their own destiny, in contrast to residents who may feel anxious, vulnerable and alone.

A REFLECTION ON THE EARLY YEARS

It is interesting to note that as far back as 1967, it was acknowledged that the care of older people was not right and that things needed to change. Rolph (1967) wrote of harrowing conditions and mistreatment, but also held the insight for what needed to happen, seeking a court of protection to protect people against physical discomfort, emotional exploitation and deprivation, using terms such as 'safeguarding'.

I am not sure that we truly knew what person-centred care was until we started practising it completely. As a care assistant in the 1980s, I knew that some of the things I saw and some of the things I was asked to do were absolutely not person-centred, but when I challenged this, it was quite obvious that I was expected to comply with a very task-orientated routine, or be deemed slow or lazy. Our main mission on the busy ward was to ensure that people were kept clean and comfortable, well fed and free from pressure sores. Patients were simply that, patients, in need of full care due to their debilitating dementia.

Most staff genuinely cared about the patients in their care, but with one member of staff to eight quite highly dependent patients, it seemed that working to a routine was the only possible option. Unfortunately, because of that routine, we would often have to battle with a patient to get them washed and dressed in time, leaving them (and the staff) exhausted and distressed. If the patient had not got any of their own clothes, replacements would be found from the 'ward stock', which were often ill-fitting.

Mealtimes were often equally chaotic, as two patients were fed in turn by one member of the care team, and then it was back to the toilet, patients lined up in wheelchairs, waiting their turn. Drinks came out on a trolley, a big teapot or milky coffee. Everybody had sugar and milk, unless they were diabetic.

Bath time took place according to the patient's scheduled day (usually seven days after their previous one), and baths took approximately eight minutes each – more of a 'sheep dip' than a pleasurable, relaxing bath time experience – but we knew the patients were clean, their hair had been washed and their nails duly clipped.

The night time routine was often dictated by how many patients the night staff had got up in the morning; we would then deliver the same number of people into their bed. The remainder of the patients would be washed and transferred into their nightwear, as we knew that the night staff had fewer resources and would be pushed for time.

Throughout the night, everybody was checked, at least every two hours, sheets were pulled back or hands went underneath the bedding to ensure that the patient had not been incontinent. If they had, they were changed and tucked back in.

This was care at its most fundamental – care that ensured everybody was clean and well fed.

BLASTS FROM THE MEDIA

Reflecting back to the early years, the care may have been fundamental, but the staff, for the most part, genuinely cared about the patients they were looking after. It was time that was a factor in restricting any further input with regard to psychological or social intervention, rather than a lack of intent.

In contrast, in 2011, we were shown the harrowing conditions at Winterbourne View (DH 2012), via a documentary that left genuine carers and trained nurses across the UK squirming in their chairs, shouting at the television and reaching for their tissues. Restraint had been used as a first-line intervention rather than as a last resort, and on occasions it had even been used for the staff's amusement.

It was abhorrent. It was ingrained and it was a culture that had been allowed to grow and develop and had obviously become the 'norm' for those staff within it. The leaders of the unit, although not directly involved in the abuse itself, had simply turned a blind eye, so yes, they were as culpable as the staff carrying out the abuse.

The general public were left aghast, some believing that this type of 'care' was widespread, and that this must have been acceptable practice. External regulators had also missed the signs, leaving many wondering how this sort of practice had been allowed to take place.

The care industry as a whole took a real hammering from the media, the public and the regulators, all of whom wanted to ensure that this sort of practice was not widespread – surely we were in an era of person-centred approaches?

Shortly after this, the Francis report was published (Francis 2013), whereby a local hospital was thoroughly investigated following numerous complaints from relatives. Restraint and ill treatment was not the focus here, but a tolerance of poor standards of care and poor communication between relevant agencies, leading to a risk for the patients.

It is little wonder, then, that the general public has become a little wary of admitting their loved ones into any healthcare facility, but there are great care homes (and hospitals) out there, places that truly follow a person-centred approach and want the very best for the resident (or patient) in their care; it is hoped that the following chapters will demonstrate how this can be achieved.

SO WHEN DID PERSON-CENTRED CARE START?

Following the introduction of the NHS and Community Care Act (1990) in the early 1990s, the large institutions that had been caring for people with mental health problems began to close down, and patients were moved into community settings.

Gone were the stark walls, the long corridors, the linoleum floors, and in their place, much smaller units, carpeted corridors, ornaments and pictures, and individual bedrooms that were homely. Some organisations moved away from traditional uniforms, another step to reduce any institutional impact. The homely feel of the new environments helped enormously in reducing the impact of a large institution, and staff could begin to see how care could be delivered differently. There was certainly a greater shift in staff thinking about the workplace as the resident's home.

It was not, however, until we went to complete a Dementia Care Mapping™ (DCM) course (University of Bradford 2005) at the University of Bradford that for those of us attending the course, we truly began to appreciate what person-centred care really meant for someone living with dementia.

Tom Kitwood was one of the course leaders. A truly inspirational man, his role-play of a person with dementia was incredible, and his insights remarkable. At that time (our group of participants trained on Edition 6), the emphasis was on how to reduce malignant social psychology (Kitwood 1997) – things that we do to people or say to people (or don't do or say), often without malice, that can often have an incredible impact on those we are caring for.

A few of us went home and became quite tearful, thinking about the times when we had unwittingly disempowered somebody or perhaps treated them like a child, when we thought we were actually helping. We had wanted to be the most caring nurses, to do everything we possibly could to help our patients, whereas in fact, for part of the time, it seems we had not helped at all.

THE MIDDLE YEARS

At the end of the 1990s, breaking into the millennium, Kitwood's work around person-centred care (1997) not only encouraged those of us who read his book to question what we were practising then, but it also gave practitioners a positive outlook to how it could be in the future.

Kitwood's writing around malignant social psychology in particular made so much sense. If we could begin to eliminate that, we could surely go forward. In addition, his approach to what we had always learned to be holistic, that was never very clear, was extremely succinct and made so much sense. We started to see the person, rather than the illness. We understood that it was not only the physical things that might affect the person, but their personality, their life story, their level of cognitive impairment and the things that were happening around them. Together, people's journeys with a diagnosis of dementia would be very different according to the interplay of the other influencing factors that accompanied the diagnosis itself.

Care plans began to take on a new life, moving away from a strictly medical model of care focusing on the dementia itself and the impact that it might have, and beginning to incorporate the other factors that may distress the person if they were not adhered to.

Company brochures and government publications began spouting their person-centred care promises, but generally, people had not fully adopted the concept of what it actually meant. As an example, the *National Service Framework for Older People* (DH 2001) dedicated one of their eight standards to person-centred care, which went some way to bridge the gap that we had been experiencing, but did not portray the things that we had been learning from Kitwood. It published that we should be promoting dignity and choice, and that services should be aligned, that health and social services staff should work together to receive a 'timely and appropriate' care package – all very good ideas, but not the essence of person-centred care.

Within the same year, the original *Essence of Care*, a patient-focused benchmarking tool (DH 2010a) was launched, comprised of ten benchmarks to improve patient care. One of these again focused on privacy and dignity, asking staff to audit their own interventions, and did start to introduce some concepts such as patients or residents not being treated as 'objects'.

My colleagues and I felt strongly, however, that the government publication, if it wanted to move to a more person-centred approach, should have a whole benchmark dedicated to person-centred care so that it ran through the other benchmarks (Baker and Edwards 2002).

At least the concepts of person-centred care were being widely talked about, in however small a way. The notion was beginning to infiltrate; people were starting to take notice.

FOUNDATIONS WITHIN THE ORGANISATION

As an organisation, Four Seasons Health Care has always been committed to providing person-centred care since I joined them in 2005, but at that time there was no dedicated training in person-centred approaches, or any thoughts about providing specialist dementia care. The company was, however, keen to listen and to provide the resources needed to make both a reality rather than just a concept.

Our journey started with 150 care homes providing care for people living with dementia. We began to deliver two-day courses, focusing on person-centred approaches for people living with dementia in our care homes. They were highly evaluated and people wanted more! It was therefore quickly agreed that we could increase the resources in the team.

We have since increased the number of care homes providing care for people living with dementia, and now have over 200 units. Our team currently comprises 24 people, 18 of whom are highly skilled practitioners working up and down the UK developing our care homes, and highly skilled administration staff help to keep it all rolling!

The person-centred courses were beginning to work, changes in practice began to occur, but reflecting back, there was still a focus on disability rather than ability – people saw 'ill-being' rather than 'well-being' opportunities. We still referred to 'challenging behaviour'.

A specific Dementia Care Manual was developed for the organisation, to help those we hadn't yet reached, to begin to implement some of the practices and interventions we spoke about. It was quite clear, though, that without the face-to-face training, people were often struggling to implement the 'new ideas'.

We began to roll out DCM training and later on, resident experience training (discussed further in Chapter 10), but it still proved difficult sometimes to consolidate and coordinate the practices and to share expert ideas. There were pockets of excellence up and down the country, but most were providing excellent essential care rather than specialist dementia care.

When I took on a new role within the company as a dedicated dementia services director, our new CEO Pete Calveley, a general practitioner (GP) by background, suggested that I put something together, a set of criteria and a pilot project that would bring all the elements of the best research and evidence-based practice that we would expect to see.

Christine Bryden (diagnosed with dementia at the age of 46) was a real inspiration to us in our work going forward (Bryden 2005). Her book talks of her journey with dementia as a dance with her partner, adjusting her steps along the way. She, too, echoed the value of Kitwood's work around person-centred care, and how important it was to her. She also talked of things that she didn't want to happen from the perspective of somebody living with dementia. These were crucial insights for us. We often cared for people in the moderate to advanced stages of dementia who were not able to explain some of the thoughts that Christine articulated. We wrote to Christine and asked if we could use some of her material to put together a training session, to which she warmly agreed.

Because we felt that Christine was such a big part of our training and our ethos, we wanted to name the programme to reflect something within Christine's book. Sharon Jones, who was working with us at that time, chose the name 'PEARL' as the references around this within Christine's book were so poignant.

> The precious string of pearls, of memories, that is our life, is breaking, the pearls are being lost. But by finding new pearls, those created in the struggle with dementia, we can put together a new necklace of life, of hope in our future. (Bryden 2005 p170)

The PEARL programme (Baker 2009) was launched in 2008, our aim to 'Positively Enrich And enhance Residents' Lives' within our dementia care units.

HOW WE PUT PERSON-CENTRED CARE INTO PRACTICE NOW

Following the pilot programme, we further developed the criteria and worked with Professor Dawn Brooker to amalgamate these into the VIPS framework (Brooker 2007).

V: A Value base that asserts the absolute value of all human lives regardless of age or cognitive ability

I: An Individualised approach, recognising uniqueness

P: Understanding the world from the Perspective of the service user

S: Providing a Social environment that supports psychological needs

PCC (person-centred care) $= V + I + P + S$

The framework gave us a clear guideline to work towards, and enabled us to align all of the policies and procedures within the same concept, giving much more relevance for us as a care home group to the idea of her model.

VIPS FRAMEWORK

How we Value people (V)

How do we value people? Valuing people must begin with valuing each other and the ethos or vision that we are working towards. Staff within the home must be person-centred with each other to enable them to be fully person-centred towards their residents. Greater emphasis is given to the role of the care worker within the dementia care setting, highlighting that it is in fact a specialist area of care. This has been strengthened by the huge focus in the media of late and the recent publications such as the *National Dementia Strategy* (DH 2009).

Throughout the programme, staff are taught to have a real empathy with those living with dementia, to try and understand how it might feel to live in a care home. They are taught to see the person and not the disease, to recognise the uniqueness of the person and their value in our society.

Within this section of the VIPS framework, we also look at how we can physically adapt the environment to help promote orientation for the residents (further explained in Chapter 9). We often ask our staff to think back to the day that they started at the home, and to remember how difficult it was on occasions to locate the treatment room or the office, and how incredibly frustrating it might be if they had short-term memory loss all of the time. Environmental cues using colour or signage can make a really big difference to reducing some of those frustrations and ultimate anxiety about being 'lost'.

Valuing can be as 'simple' as using somebody's name, their preferred form of address rather than a term of endearment, such as 'love' or 'pet'. We know for ourselves that if we return to a restaurant and they remember our name, or even something about us, we feel as if we are valued customers. This should be no different for a resident living in a care home.

One of the key messages within the V section of the framework is that the value applies to all, to residents, to staff, and to their friends or relatives. Valuing is primarily about involving, respecting, increasing knowledge and treating everybody as an equal.

How we apply an Individualised approach (I)

Some may say that it is difficult to adopt a truly individualised approach within a care environment, but this is simply not true. It can take some considerable time to make the switch from a task-focused routine to a person-centred routine as all the staff need to be understand why they are making the change, particularly if the home is fairly 'set in its ways'. Staff have told me that it would take many more staff to deliver care in such an individual way, but what they don't realise, until we do the training, is that often residents become resistant to care when it isn't tailored to their individual needs. Residents then become anxious and distressed, which is dreadful for them, frustrating for the staff and much more time-consuming than working out how we can provide individual care for individual needs.

Stepping out into person-centred approaches can be a bit like juggling plates, and can feel a bit uncomfortable for staff. They have felt nurtured by their own routines, safe in the knowledge that all baths have been done, the tea round complete, people tucked into bed.

We can still make all of those things happen, but not necessarily at the same time as everybody else! We only have to think about ourselves and how our days differ, from the time we get up, have our breakfast (and what do we eat) to what we do with ourselves in the day. We are not all the same and we therefore cannot expect that our residents will conform to a routine because it is easier for us. It is their home, not ours.

Life story work has been key to our programme, helping staff to appreciate how things the resident has experienced, albeit positive or negative, can have an enormous impact on their levels of well-being and the reduction of distress (further explained in Chapter 3).

It can be difficult to determine sometimes what a person really needs if they are not able to tell us. In this section of the VIPS framework we also explore how staff can begin to unpick the signs that they are seeing, using specialist observational tools to determine if residents may be in pain or perhaps depressed (further explained in Chapter 11).

Individualised approaches in the context of Brooker's model also apply to the level and type of activity that the resident might want to engage in (further explained in Chapter 9), a crucial factor for many within a dementia care home.

How we understand the world from the Perspective of the resident (P)

At first glance, this section of the framework appears a bit more difficult to tackle, particularly if like most of our care homes, people are in the moderate to advanced stages of their journey with dementia, and may find it difficult to verbally express their needs. This is when staff can have a tendency to 'take over', to make assumptions, to ask the resident but not wait for an answer.

Keen observation is paramount in a dementia care setting. Often, the residents do communicate with us in a non-verbal way. When we get to know our residents really well, we can tell when they are happy or sad, if they are in pain, if they are thirsty, if they are tired.

DCM has been a really useful tool (further explained in Chapters 2 and 10) in helping us to assess and evaluate the care that the resident is receiving, and helping us to relay this to the staff working within the unit so that we can all focus on improving the person's level of well-being.

When the resident does tell us what they need, we need to listen! We must not assume that the resident is unable to make a meaningful decision because of cognitive impairment.

Through our programme, we encourage staff to work with residents in a proactive way, to try and interpret any potential difficulties before they might arise, to 'read' the non-verbal signs or vocalisations, acting before the resident might become distressed (further explained in Chapter 7).

The perspective of the resident is crucial to person-centred care. If we struggle to get our approaches or timing right, we can potentially damage the resident's level of well-being, often unknowingly or unwittingly inducing ill-being.

How we provide a Social environment that supports psychological needs (S)

We have a real focus on this area within our homes. Prior to us implementing the programme, our environments could be quite noisy and residents could be seen walking around, sometimes seemingly without a sense of purpose. At times they appeared lost, distressed, and anxious.

Today we have environments that encourage activity, that help residents to find their way around. We look at what may present as a risk, and try and eliminate that as far as we can, and we encourage our staff to treat every intervention as an activity and not simply a procedure.

Our CEO went to all of the homes involved in the pilot project before and after the programme, and he was astonished by the difference in the environment and how calm it subsequently felt.

A large part of this section of the framework is also looking at the reduction of the malignant social psychology I spoke about earlier – educating staff about the adverse effects of disempowering, talking over residents' heads or perhaps carrying out an intervention that is too quick for residents to fully process what is happening to them or around them.

A supportive social environment focuses on the involvement of residents with the day-to-day running of the care home, and how we can facilitate and maintain their connections with their community.

PERSON-CENTRED CARE SHOULD BE NATURAL!

For all that is written about person-centred care, it really is very simple to deliver! All staff really need to do is to question themselves about how they themselves would want to receive care as a starting point, and what might upset them and what would happen if this varied from their expectations. They need to appreciate how this might feel for them, and how this also applies to the feelings of the residents in our care. They need to involve the person receiving care (and their friend or relative, if that helps), and carry out the care according to the person's wishes.

There are obviously occasions when we need to make a 'best interest' decision (Mental Capacity Act 2005), but for the most part, if we work with the resident in the way that the resident wishes to be cared for, we will have a winning formula.

Chapter 2

Nothing About Me Without Me

In this chapter, I describe how we can try to involve the person living with dementia in the care home to help them to reach decisions about the care that they would like to receive. Gone, thankfully, are the days that we 'do for' and 'at' people living with dementia. Even for those who are in the advancing stages of their diagnosis, it is still possible to try and elicit their views of how they would like to receive their care through enhanced communication skills and specialist tools such as Dementia Care Mapping™ (DCM). This chapter also looks at the Mental Capacity Act 2005, and at how it can assist us in providing care for residents who may lack capacity.

The phrase 'Nothing About Me Without Me' was coined within a government paper that refreshingly stated that 'patients will be at the heart of everything we do' (DH 2010b, p.1). A great concept, and one that we should all be following.

Historically, decision making was taken away from people with a cognitive impairment as there was a real fear that they may make the 'wrong decision'. Other reasons cited were that the person might become frustrated trying to make a decision if given a choice.

Further compounding this was a real difficulty if people were also not able to verbally communicate – surely they were not able to make a decision?

Thankfully, the thinking around inclusion, giving people a voice (and a choice) has improved dramatically over the past few years, and the Mental Capacity Act 2005 has supported us to do this. External regulators across the UK are now asking for evidence of resident and relative involvement within the care planning process, although this does not always prove easy to achieve, particularly if the resident has advanced cognitive impairment and does not have a close relative. If a relative is involved but the resident lacks capacity to consent, how we can be sure that the resident would want the relative to view the contents of their care plan? This is a real ethical dilemma, one that promotes much discussion within our care homes.

HOW CAN WE INCLUDE RESIDENTS IN THE CARE HOME?

At its most simple level, we really should be asking our residents what they would like to happen, what they need and when they are most likely to need it. As care professionals we need to look at ourselves and at how we communicate to ensure that we are giving residents time to process the information that we are asking, time to formulate a response, and finally, to respond to our question.

Staff are often busy in the care home, rushing around, conscious of the next thing that they need to do, and so often they will ask residents a question, and try to involve them, but when there is not an immediate response, they will either take the decision for them or carry on to their next job.

This is mainly down to the carer's confidence, and to a certain extent, their knowledge. If staff do not realise how dementia can affect the communication process, they may struggle to understand why they might not get an immediate response. Of course, when looking at this in a harsh light, it may be that the carer chooses to carry on regardless because they do not have time to wait for a response, or deem that the person will not be able to give an informative answer.

WHAT IF THE ANSWER IS NOT ONE THAT WE WOULD EXPECT?

Sometimes, it can be really difficult to ask the question because we are worried that the answer is not one that we might want to hear.

As an example, we base a scenario on 'Harry'. We want to encourage Harry to visit the toilet as we know that he has not been for a couple of hours. We ask him if he would like to use the toilet, we wait, and he responds 'No.' What do we do now?!

This is where 'best interest' decisions begin to form part of our process, but for now, I will look at the stance of a person-centred approach, looking for signs of well-being.

Scenario 1

Our resident, Harry, has clearly told me that he doesn't want to use the toilet. He doesn't look uncomfortable or distressed, and therefore I make the assumption that he is in a level of well-being, that he is being assertive and quite clear about his decision. I therefore respect his decision and communicate to him that this is fine and I will come back to him later. I continue to observe him to ensure that he is still comfortable and showing no signs of ill-being.

Scenario 2

Harry has clearly told me that he doesn't want to use the toilet but he looks uncomfortable, he is fidgeting and looking slightly distressed. I suspect that he may need to go to the toilet but is unable to relay this to me at the current time. I again respect his decision, and tell him I will be back shortly. When I return a few minutes later, I rephrase my communication. I am aware that Harry really needs to visit the toilet and I am aware that he said no last time. I don't want to disempower Harry or ignore his choice and so this time, I do not offer a choice. This is because I know that Harry needs to go to the toilet and to continue to respect his decision, given that he looks so uncomfortable, would not be person-centred or helpful to Harry. I have made an informal best interest decision.

This may take the form of 'Hello Harry, let's pop along to the toilet.' I am therefore giving a kind instruction rather than offering a choice in this case. If we know that this would be a regular occurrence for Harry, we should incorporate this into his care plan so that all staff know how to communicate with Harry when he needs the toilet.

Within the scenario, we find that Harry responds well to us using kind directional communication and will happily go to the toilet but sometimes, even using effective communication and person-centred approaches does not always resolve a situation.

USING THE MENTAL CAPACITY ACT 2005

The Mental Capacity Act is quite complex, and readers will need to read the full Code of Practice to enable them to fully appreciate and understand its use and application to care delivery.

To enable readers to relate to the use of the Act in practice, I use a scenario of a situation for a resident we come across quite often in our care homes. For this scenario, we will look at 'Phoebe'.

Scenario 3

Phoebe has been in the care home for a couple of years. She has always taken her medication really well and was often heard to comment in the initial few months that her medication always helped her to feel better. Her husband, George, informed us that Phoebe religiously took her medication at the same time each day, and would become quite anxious if she thought it was going to be late. He said that she had always been to visit the doctor if she was worried about anything, and believed that 'the doctor knew best' and would take any medication prescribed to her. Phoebe needs to take blood-thinning medication along with medication to help her with her diabetes.

During the last couple of days, Phoebe has been reluctant to take her medication. Staff have tried to coax her and to gently explain why she needs to take her medication, but she is either not taking them, or removing the tablets from her mouth.

Staff are concerned that Phoebe may become ill if she does not take her medication, and so they contact the general practitioner (GP). The GP suggests that they give her the medication covertly as she really needs to take it.

CARRYING OUT A CAPACITY ASSESSMENT

Initially, the staff would carry out a capacity assessment, and this must be decision-specific, that is, the need to take medication covertly. First, the staff would establish if Phoebe has a form of cognitive impairment that may make it difficult for her to make an independent decision. This is referred to as Stage 1 of the Mental Capacity Act.

Within Stage 2 of the capacity assessment, staff would then establish if the cognitive impairment would render Phoebe unable to make a decision about taking her medication covertly (in this instance).

It is critical that staff use everything they can draw on to help Phoebe to be involved in and to communicate her decision. Staff should speak clearly, and wait for a response. Staff can use pictures or large print if this would help. There has also been research to show that Talking Mats (Murphy, Oliver and Cox 2010) can assist people living with dementia in the early to moderate stages to make a decision, and these are used within some of our care homes. Staff must also ensure that they approach the resident at a time when it may be 'easier' for them to make a decision. For example, if we know a resident appears quite lucid in the morning but becomes more confused as the day goes on, we would make sure that we carried out the assessment in the morning.

Questions we would then consider when carrying out the assessment would be:

1. Does the resident understand the information relevant to the decision?

2. Is the resident able to retain the information long enough to make a decision?

3. Is the resident able to use or weigh that information as part of the process of making the decision?

4. Is the resident able to communicate their decision (whether by speech, sign language or any other means)?

We will assume for this scenario that Phoebe is unable to make any decision. However, it is important that we don't simply put 'no' in response to these questions if we are to demonstrate a comprehensive assessment. We should document how Phoebe reacted, what we saw, what we heard, what we used to help us to reach our decision.

Once we are fully satisfied that Phoebe lacks the capacity to make a decision, we then need to make a best interest decision.

HOW DO WE MAKE A BEST INTEREST DECISION?

The staff, George (the husband), the GP and the pharmacist need to reach a best interest decision (Mental Capacity Act 2005) for Phoebe to receive her medication covertly.

The staff would complete the best interest checklist (as described in the Code of Practice in the Mental Capacity Act 2005) in conjunction with George, her GP and the pharmacist where possible. Although it may not be possible to bring everybody together at the same time, the same questions should be asked to establish that all parties are in agreement.

Resident's Name: Phoebe   D.O.B: XX/XX/XXXX

Nature of Decision: *(Record in the space below the specific decision for which the resident lacks capacity)*

Accepting medication covertly

Checklist *(please highlight the appropriate answer and add any comments in as much detail as possible in support of evidence for the decision)*

1 Is there an advance decision made by the resident to refuse specified medical treatment which is valid and applicable to current circumstances?

Complete the rest of the checklist only if the answer is NO

YES / NO

2 Are you satisfied that the assessment of best interests is not based simply on the resident's age, appearance, condition or behaviour?

YES / NO

3 Is the treatment urgent and therefore it is not practicable to delay making the decision until the resident regains capacity?

YES / NO

4 Has every effort been made to encourage and enable the resident to take part in making the decision?

YES / NO

5 Have you identified and considered all relevant circumstances that the resident would take into account if they were making the decision for themselves?

YES / NO

6 Are you taking into account the resident's past and present wishes and feelings (these may have been expressed verbally, in writing or through behaviour or habits)?

YES / NO

7 Have you considered any beliefs and values (e.g. religious, cultural, moral or political) that would be likely to influence the resident's decision if they were making it themselves?

YES / NO

8 Have you considered other options and alternative actions that may be less restrictive of the resident's rights?

YES / NO

9 For life-sustaining treatment, are you fully satisfied that the decision is not motivated in any way by a desire to bring about the resident's death?

YES / NO

10 Have you consulted other people for their views about the resident's best interests and for any information about their wishes and feelings, beliefs and values?

Anyone previously named by the person in advance as someone to be consulted?

YES / NO   Name: Contact No:

Any relatives, friends or others who take an interest in the person's welfare?

YES / NO   Name: Contact No:

Anyone engaged in caring for the person?

YES / NO   Name: Contact No:

Any attorney appointed under a Lasting Power of Attorney or Enduring Power of Attorney?

YES / NO   Name: Contact No:

Any deputy appointed by the Court of Protection to make decisions for the person?

YES / NO   Name: Contact No:

For decisions about serious medical treatment and longer-term accommodation/placement, where there is no one to consult, an independent mental capacity advocate (IMCA) MUST be consulted.

Any other relevant information or particular factors taken into account whilst making the decision.

Signed ....

Date ....

Name ....

Position ....

Figure 2.1: Best interest checklist for resident lacking capacity

The first three areas within the best interest checklist ensure that we are not making our judgements on age, appearance, condition or behaviour alone, that we have considered an advanced decision if there is one in place, and if the treatment is urgent.

Given that Phoebe has not taken her medication and it may adversely affect her if she misses any further doses, this would be deemed as urgent. We do not know of any advanced decision in place and her age, appearance, condition or behaviour has not influenced our assessment or thoughts around why she should receive medication covertly.

The fourth area asks the assessor to ensure that they have made every effort to encourage and enable the resident to take part in making the decision. Staff in this particular scenario would have ensured that they had spoken to Phoebe about the importance of her medication, they would have used non-verbal cues such as presenting the medication at the time it was due, reassuring Phoebe that she had always taken her medication in the past. Staff would have returned with the medication at a later time to offer the medication again. During the capacity assessment itself, staff would have also discussed this and would also have ascertained if Phoebe was able to understand the importance of not taking the medication and the issues that may arise.

The fifth, sixth and seventh areas are most significant here for this particular scenario, namely:

- that we consider all the relevant circumstances residents would take into account if they were making the decision for themselves

- that we take into account the resident's past and present wishes and feelings

- that we consider any beliefs and values that would be likely to influence the resident's decision if they were making it themselves.

In this particular scenario, George has been able to tell us about Phoebe's feelings around taking medication prior to developing a cognitive impairment. When we re-visit the information that he has given us, he is absolutely clear that Phoebe, if she had capacity, would be taking her medication, and is fully behind the best interest decision to give the medication covertly.

Phoebe's GP was able to back this up, confirming that Phoebe readily accepted what he had told her in the past, and that she never hesitated to take her medication and that she had, in fact, phoned him on a couple of occasions when she had accidently forgotten a dose to make sure that she would be okay. He therefore felt that it was in Phoebe's best interest to receive her medication covertly.

The pharmacist was also supportive of the decision, as he knew that when Phoebe lived at home, she would make absolutely sure that she had enough medication for the coming weeks. The pharmacist confirmed that both types of medication that Phoebe was receiving could be 'crushed' safely.

The care team working with Phoebe were all concerned that she was not taking her medication, and although they didn't particularly want to 'hide' her medication in order for her to take it, they realised that it was really important for her to have it and therefore also agreed to the best interest decision.

The eighth area asks us if we have considered other options and alternative actions that may be less restrictive of the resident's rights. In this particular scenario, this would be considered the least restrictive, as without the intervention decided on, Phoebe may have to be admitted to hospital.

Area nine considers the notion that for life-sustaining treatment, as a decision-making group, we are fully satisfied that the decision is not motivated in any way by a desire to bring about the resident's death. Again, in this scenario, we can be confident that the opposite is true. We are taking the decision to maintain or improve Phoebe's physical condition.

In the final area, the checklist asks us to review whether or not we have consulted others for any information about Phoebe's wishes and feelings, beliefs and values. Staff would then review and document a summary of the discussion and the subsequent decision and who was involved, and document this into Phoebe's care plan.

CHANGE CAN HAPPEN OVERNIGHT

Whilst every care has been taken to ensure that Phoebe has had a best interest decision taken for her, we must remember that situations and people can change overnight through their journey with dementia, and as such, staff must ensure that the current decision is the most suitable one for the resident. It may be that Phoebe will start taking her medication again independently, and we should periodically try to offer the medication in the usual way, rather than covertly.

HOW CAN RELATIVES OR FRIENDS HELP US TO SUPPORT THE RESIDENT?

The information that George provided regarding Phoebe was really useful and helped enormously in reaching a best interest decision. It is so important that we try and record the wishes of people living with dementia before their dementia diagnosis advances as we can use any information that they have documented to support any best interest decision going forward.

Even prior to admission, we should try and establish key facts about the person's life story, wishes, likes and dislikes so that we are better prepared for the person coming into the home and can begin to formulate care plans that have real meaning and focus (more on this in Chapters 3 and 4).

If we are not able to elicit any information from the resident prior to or following admission, the care staff should talk to the relative or friend of the person as soon as possible to establish how the person might prefer to receive care, or how the care provided by them has worked well and, equally as important, what hasn't worked well.

It is important that the relative or friend is not excluded, even if residents are able to give us information for themselves, as relatives often want to be and feel part of the process. They have often been looking after the person at home for some considerable time.

The relative or friend should (if the resident consents and the relative agrees) be an equal part of the admission process. No member of staff will ever know the resident as well as they do if they have been the full-time carer for the person prior to them coming to the care home. This doesn't mean to say that different approaches cannot be tried, but it is important to include the relative or friend in the thoughts around the new ideas or approaches so that they can offer their own ideas and be part of the planning process.

Specifically, with regard to best interest decisions, the relative or friend may help the staff to work through a process to establish if the resident 'may have done something or not done something' prior to their diagnosis. For example, if a resident really enjoys walking around the home but is at risk of falls, staff may be concerned and continually encourage the person to remain seated. By talking to the relative, it gives both parties an opportunity to discuss this, and how it may affect the person's overall well-being. Would the resident be more upset about being asked to sit down or be more upset if they fell and injured themself? What we think and do, generally, to protect our residents, is not necessarily what residents would choose to do if they had full capacity.

HOW CAN DEMENTIA CARE MAPPING™ HELP US WITHIN THE CARE HOME?

In brief, Dementia Care Mapping™ (DCM) (University of Bradford 2005) is a specialist observational tool that allows us to look at the things that people living with dementia in our care home are doing, how they are responding to the particular activity, and how staff interactions may affect this, in either a positive or negative way.

We currently have over 500 staff trained in DCM working within our care homes. DCM for us is used as an analytical tool and a way of helping to design bespoke training and person-centred plans rather than a strict measurement of well-being, although it is also used by our Dementia Care Services Team to validate the care being given within our specialist units.

A person trained in DCM will discreetly observe up to six residents, taking note of the type of behaviour they are engaged in, for example, eating and drinking, taking part in a leisure activity or walking up and down. They will then look at the resident's mood and engagement level during the activity – is it a positive mood and engagement state or is the resident experiencing a negative mood or engagement state? This judgement is carried out at the end of every five minutes. Alongside this, the mapper categorises the interventions carried out by the staff – are they good (enhancing) or not so good (detracting), and did they affect the resident's mood or engagement level?

This way, if a resident is not able to verbally tell us how they are experiencing care, we are able to build a picture of what works well for the resident, what they appear to enjoy and what they do not want to happen. All of this information can be included within residents' assessments and subsequent care plans when the information is fed back to the staff.

WHAT OTHER TOOLS CAN WE USE TO HELP US TO INVOLVE THE RESIDENT?

Our biggest tool is our vision! When working in a dementia care setting it is often what we see rather than what we hear that will help to guide us to the needs of the resident. That doesn't mean to say that we don't listen to the residents; of course we do, but often, observation of the more subtle non-verbal communication gives a much bigger picture.

When we get to know our residents really well, we can see when they appear to be tired, hungry, in pain, restless, or wanting to get up and explore. We can see when the resident sitting next door to them is beginning to cause some distress, and they are then asked if they would like to spend some time in the garden or in their room so that they can have some relaxation.

Sometimes talking around a subject can help a resident to offer their views rather than direct questioning. I have often found that a resident will offer their opinion on something in 'general conversation', but it is important that we capture those thoughts and record them in their assessment or care plan so that all staff are aware.

Pictures can often help to facilitate conversations or help residents to make a choice, for example, showing a resident a picture of the various meals on offer enabling them to make a choice or during mealtimes – showing the resident the choices of the actual meals on offer for them to make a selection.

EVERY DECISION IN EVERYDAY CARE

Involving residents is not only about the big decisions we need to take in life. It revolves around everyday decisions, all of the time. Everything we do should be done in consultation with the resident we are caring for, seeking their consent, establishing their preference and promoting their abilities where we can.

Chapter 3

Life Story and Lifestyle

In this chapter, I explore how our life story shapes the people we are, and how parts of our life story are critical to how we may want (or not want) to receive care. This chapter describes ways in which we might gather life story information and, equally as important, how we might transfer the knowledge into everyday care.

We need to find the pearl hidden within us. Like the pearl that is formed through the irritation of a grain of sand within an oyster, our pearl has formed through the challenge of living with dementia. Finding this pearl within is the key to creating a new future of life in the slow lane. (Bryden 2005 p.168)

WHY IS LIFE STORY AND LIFESTYLE SO IMPORTANT?

Everybody has a story to tell, and some of the things that happen to us during our lifetime may affect us either in the current moment or later in life, be those positive or negative experiences or memories.

In dementia care, it is particularly important to look at memories and experiences that may have occurred many years ago as the person's short-term memory fades or becomes lost.

What happens in the present moment may also remind a person of their past (or someone significant from their past), and we have to acknowledge and work with the resident within their frame of reference.

As well as life stories, we also need to appreciate the resident's roles prior to them coming into the care home as they may well have a great influence on the way they experience their care.

A resident coming into the care home may have had many roles prior to their admission – a wife, a husband, a mother, a father, a grandmother, a sister, a brother, a former teacher. The lived experience in the care home may vary for each resident, dependent on the memories they are re-living at any given time. Our key strength as care providers is to work with, rather than against, the person's experience.

We often see residents reverting to their former roles within the care home, for example, a former postman who got up very early every day, going round to residents' rooms and knocking on their doors. Sometimes it is not always practical to work alongside the resident, as in this case – it would disturb other residents within the home. What we can do is draw on aspects of the role itself and encourage the resident to help us to sort through some post and help us to make a decision as to where it will go, for example, and use the time with the resident to talk about their former role and experience of it.

I remember a headmistress in one of our homes who constantly 'told the other residents off', telling them to behave and to sit down and be quiet, as she believed she was still in her role within the school, and the residents before her were her children. Because we knew this about this particular lady, we were able to work alongside her and guide her into other activities that occupied her frame of reference at that time, encouraging her to look at 'registers', at the diary or at some books. This helped her to feel that she was doing something of value, which ultimately maintained her well-being and self-esteem, and reduced the risk of distress for the other residents within the care home.

We have other residents who have worked in offices who enjoy sitting in the manager's office helping them to file, and residents who had previously worked in the gardens helping the gardener, although we do also have some residents who make it quite plain that they have now retired, and no longer want to be involved, thank you!

Within our homes, all of our staff are encouraged to take an active part in improving the residents' day and to facilitate activity. This includes the maintenance man who meets with a resident (a former engineer) for a coffee in their office before taking the resident around with them and allocating 'minimal risk' tasks that the resident can help him with. The resident who worked in a hospital laundry helps to fold the warm towels as they come out of the tumble dryer and accompanies the laundress to the rooms to take around the baskets of clothes.

Role continuity can be critical in helping to maintain a person's well-being and to give them a sense of feeling needed and able to continue as they once were. Our residents with a diagnosis of dementia will ultimately lose many skills and memories as their journey progresses; it is therefore our role to ensure that we facilitate those things that residents are still able to continue whilst they can.

When we first begin to talk to our care staff about the idea of role continuity, some are apprehensive as they are genuinely concerned that the resident may come to harm if they are not fully able to carry out a task, or if the resident forgets part-way through a task. Most of our role continuity activities are shared tasks, however, whereby the care worker can work alongside the resident to enable and facilitate, and to minimise any risk.

One of our residents who lived in a home in Scotland really missed being able to iron. Staff were understandably nervous about this, but the home's maintenance man permanently fixed the dial on a domestic iron so that it was warm but could not get hot, and the lady spent hours ironing the napkins and tea cloths. She was genuinely delighted when staff offered praise for a job well done. In this particular case, this really helped the resident to feel part of the home environment and that she was part of 'the team'.

Life story case study: 'Doreen'

On a recent visit to a care home to deliver training, the staff asked me if I could offer any advice regarding a lady who had been experiencing some distress over the past few months. Doreen, a lady in her late eighties, had been a resident in the home for the past two years.

Within her initial admission notes, it stated that Doreen could become anxious and preferred that her bedroom door was kept open. The notes gave lots of rich information about Doreen's preferences and choices and guidance on the types of interventions that may help to reduce her anxiety.

Latterly, Doreen had been observed vocalising, with no apparent trigger. She had been admitted to general hospital a few months prior to my visit following a fall, resulting in a fractured neck of femur. She had been prescribed strong pain relief, which she continued to take, an anti-depressant and medication to reduce her anxiety.

Staff had tried various interventions to reduce her anxiety, and had also involved the local clinical psychologist, consultant psychiatrist and community mental health nurse. Following these visits, further medication was prescribed to see if this would help reduce Doreen's anxiety level.

As I entered Doreen's room prior to meeting her, I noticed that her room was full of personal memorabilia, lots of pictures of her (quite expansive) family, photo albums, personal effects from her home, and the room generally had a nice homely feel. I read her life story summary and noted Doreen's previous occupation and some key information about her life before I went down to introduce myself.

I met Doreen in the main lounge of the care home. She appeared quite distressed and as the staff had reported, she was calling out, nothing of note, but appeared quite anxious.

I initially knelt down beside her and began to talk to her, and observed that she continued to call out. We asked if she would like to accompany us to her room, and after some initial hesitation, she got up from her chair and walked with us to her bedroom.

Doreen was communicating to us as we walked, but continued to 'cry out' intermittently. I noticed that she did seem quite stiff when she first started to mobilise, and wondered if perhaps her pain relief needed to be increased. However, as we progressed along the corridor, she mobilised quite easily, but continued to call out.

As we got to her room, she started to point things out to me on her dressing table, and then focused on a picture of her father. She began to talk about him, commenting on his clothing, and repeatedly said 'that's my father'.

As Doreen sat down, she continued to look anxious and distressed, and as I sat beside her, continued to vocalise.

I took the picture from the dressing table and handed it to Doreen, asking her to tell me more about her father. She was unable to articulate any details to me but repeatedly said, 'my father, my father, he had to go away'. I asked Doreen if she missed her father and she disregarded my question and pointed to items of clothing that her father was wearing, providing a description of his attire. She placed the photograph in front of her on her table and continued to say 'my father, my father'. Any attempts to discover more information or to empathise or validate were disregarded, so I just stayed by Doreen's side and let her describe her father's attire whilst I listened.

After a while, I retrieved a photo album that was also on the dresser and had obviously been well used. Doreen proceeded to open the book and began to look at the various pictures within it, several of which were pictures of her father. She spent a small amount of time describing the other people depicted on the pages, but constantly came back to any pictures of her father, again lamenting 'my father, my father'.

Doreen passed the photo album back to me and again began to focus on the picture on the table, but her anxiety and distress had noticeably decreased. She began to take note of my hair and my eyes, telling me that I looked like her sister. Periodically, she would look at the picture and repeat the same comments, but the vocalisations had stopped.

She went on to say that she didn't know where she was. Her missing father was almost certainly the key to her grief; she seemed to need him around her for reassurance. It was almost as if by placing the photograph in front of her, it was helping her to feel safe. She began to listen to our reassurances of where she was and why she was there, and she visibly relaxed, which enabled us to talk to her about why she felt upset, which in the main was because she couldn't remember where she was or why she was there, but she seemed quite quickly reassured when she was able to focus fully. On reviewing Doreen's notes again following our meeting, I came across a specialist assessment by an external health agency. The assessment had asked her to make up a sentence and write it in the space below. Doreen had written 'father'.

When staff spoke to Doreen's relatives later that day, it transpired that Doreen's father had died suddenly in his early fifties.

This case study demonstrates that life story information and precious memorabilia can be invaluable in helping to reduce a resident's anxiety and distress as well as improving well-being. Staff were advised to include this intervention in Doreen's care plan, that is, to place the picture of Doreen's father in her hands in times of distress, or in front of her to help to reduce her anxiety to enable staff to talk to her about her underlying concern once her anxiety had decreased a little.

HOW CAN WE BEGIN TO GATHER INFORMATION?

There are many varied and creative ways that we have observed life stories to be gathered and presented. Life story information gathering can be a wonderful activity and opportunity for staff to develop stronger relationships with both the resident and the resident's family or friends.

We have found that relatives often want to be involved with compiling the information, and many of our relatives have produced beautiful life story books and story boards, and have found that this helped them with their own feelings about the resident's transition into full-time care.

Audio recordings

I was fortunate to be able to witness Jim Ellis (2002) with his wife Margaret many years ago. Jim had made a tape recording of his own narrative describing a holiday he had taken with Margaret. I happened to be at the home carrying out a DCM observation (University of Bradford 2005), and I was therefore able to observe Margaret's response when she listened to the tape. I observed her showing great signs of well-being. She was smiling, laughing at times, looking 'curious' at times as if she were trying to recall the particular memory that she was listening to. Jim allowed me to listen to part of the tape after I had finished my observation, and I felt privileged that I had been permitted to have a glimpse into the life that they had once shared. Jim began by taking Margaret through the ritual of packing her case, detailing how many pairs of shoes she would take and which were her favourites and why. He described them walking down the path together to the car, full of excitement at the week ahead. He then went on to provide a rich and colourful story of their week spent on their holiday.

Former studies on simulated presence therapy to meet attachment needs of people living with dementia carried out by Cheston and Byatt (1999) also showed that a resident who constantly walked around the unit would remain seated for periods of up to 35 minutes when listening to a tape of her husband talking to her. She also appeared to take much more notice of her environment and showed concern for others whilst the tape was playing.

DVDs

Visual media can really bring life stories to the forefront. One of the care homes in the North worked with the residents and their families to provide narratives, music and pictures together on a DVD. The pictures were of the residents themselves, their families, or items or objects relating to their life stories and their hobbies or work. The music playing in the background was a selection of tracks that the resident had particularly favoured during their life. The DVDs were then used either by the residents themselves or as a joint activity with either the staff or family.

Memory boxes

Within the homes, the care staff work with the residents and their families to put together individual 'portable' memory boxes. The homes did pilot the memory boxes that could be attached to the wall outside of the residents' rooms, but there was general concern around accessibility of the person's precious memorabilia. Although the wall-mounted boxes could be really useful for providing an orientation cue, residents wanted access to the things that helped to define them, to pick the boxes up, to smell them, to feel them near them. With a portable box (usually a shoe box decorated with nice paper!), the box could then be transported to the resident if they were in the lounge, for example, or passed across to them if they were in bed.

The individual memory boxes are just that, very individual, and no content will be the same. Some of the residents have copies of their birth certificates or qualifications, some boxes contain first baby shoes or pieces of lace that formed part of their wedding dress. Without doubt, all the boxes bring joy to those who hold them; sometimes there is no need for words as residents will want to sift through and select items that are precious to them, but equally, the memory boxes can be a great opportunity to discuss aspects of the person's life story.

Digital frames

Digital frames can be used within or outside of the resident's room (to act as an orientation cue). They can be uploaded with hundreds of pictures running on a 'slideshow'. Digital frames can be particularly useful, as the resident does not have to physically hold any material. For a resident who needs to be nursed in bed, the range of pictures can provide stimulation if placed on the locker by their side, and act as comfort that their family are still near.

Photo albums

It is hard to beat the 'old fashioned' photograph album, a book of sometimes random photographs, dates and names written underneath that the resident is able to thumb through at their leisure. Looking through an album together can also be a useful activity for staff to complete with the resident, as it will provide lots of opportunity for the staff to facilitate conversation around a given picture. It is always helpful if the family can provide names underneath the picture and perhaps the location where it was taken to enable the staff to use this as a cue if the resident is unable to remember.

Story boards

Some relatives have provided extremely creative story boards with family trees depicted on them, career paths, favourite quotes, etc. We have seen some huge boards in residents' rooms whereby the family tree has been drawn on it, with pictures of the relevant family on the tree. Some boards have shown a 'life path', depicting significant events through pictures and words. Some are collages of significant people in the resident's life, but all are really helpful to engage the resident in conversation.

A4 life story summaries

Within our homes, we encourage relatives to help us to provide A4 size life story summaries that we frame and put outside of the resident's door. These summaries do not contain any confidential information, but provide some key information to enable any visiting professional or new staff to familiarise themselves with a 'potted' history of the resident prior to entering their room.

Example of a life story summary: Sarah Brown's story

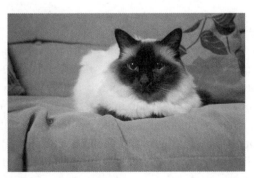

Figure 3.1: Sarah Brown's cat, Jasper

Sarah is really fond of cats – this is a picture of her favourite cat, Jasper.

Sarah was born on May 20th in Grimsby, Lincolnshire, to Terence and Margaret. Her grandfather Eddie was a fish merchant, and she enjoys eating fish, especially smoked haddock and crab.

Sarah has a brother and a sister, Audrey and Tom, who both still live in Grimsby. Audrey and Tom do not come to visit very often, as it is too far for them to travel, but they write to her regularly; Sarah enjoys having their letters read out to her. Sarah's husband Peter visits most days, and her children Charlie, Michael and Rebecca visit every Sunday. It is a real treat for Sarah if her grandchildren Alice and Geoffrey come too.

Sarah was very proud of her home and liked to keep it nice and clean and tidy. She particularly enjoyed polishing and dusting, as she used to be a cleaner in her younger days. Sarah loves to help with jobs such as making her bed and dusting her furniture.

Sarah enjoys listening to peaceful music, and watching cookery programmes on the television, as she used to be a really good cook. She enjoys baking, and likes to make cakes for her grandchildren when they come to visit.

Sarah also enjoys sitting in the garden, especially if it is a nice sunny day. She loves to chat to people over a cup of tea (and a chocolate biscuit!). Sarah takes milk and no sugar in her tea, and occasionally enjoys a coffee with milk and two sugars.

Where the life story summaries have been used we have found that not only do the staff know the residents really well, but that some residents and relatives have also made connections to each other.

Music to facilitate life stories

Music can be used in many different ways when working with people living with dementia. It can be a real catalyst to provoke memories and for staff to capture the essence of the resident's emotion and to work with them to tell their story.

Life stories through a music medium can either be used as an individual activity or within a small group, as sometimes one person's memory of an event will encourage others within the group to recall a story of their own relating to the piece of music.

LIFE STORY AS A NAVIGATION TOOL

Life story work is crucial, and central, to all of the work that we do within the care home if we are going to provide a really good experience for the resident living with dementia. It underpins our care plans, our communication and our interventions, dependent on the needs of the resident.

It can take some considerable time to gather the information that is needed, but it is undoubtedly time well spent, as time spent in the beginning will pave the way for a smoother journey, showing us (the care team) the direction to follow.

Chapter 4

Person-centred Planning

In this chapter, I consider the true meaning of a person-centred plan and how it differs from a traditional care plan. This chapter has been written to help staff and relatives/friends to put together care plans with meaning, that are achievable and that will truly help the person living with dementia in the care home environment using life story work.

As nursing students in the mid-1980s, we were shown how to write truly exceptional care plans, care plans that had wonderful goals, and very prescriptive steps, but were unfortunately not very realistic (regarding the goals), and the steps could have applied to any number of people we were caring for.

Mason (1999) describes a nursing care plan as a written, structured plan of action for patient care based on holistic assessment of patient needs, identification of specific patient problems and a development of a plan of action to provide a resolution.

Care plans were designed to inform the nurse who was working on a particular shift of the exact steps to be carried out to ensure continuous care for a patient. This has not changed.

Generally, however, the steps of the care plan were very 'woolly', a purposeful instruction from the tutors of the day so that the nurse did not land herself in hot water! A stark contrast to today, whereby specific outcomes are expected, and steps within the plan need to be very detailed with measurable results, as well as being person-centred.

A review of recent journal literature has shown very little in regards to the person-centred care planning process with the exception of care planning for people living with dementia at the end of their life. It is therefore timely that this chapter explores the importance of introducing person-centred planning into dementia care.

During the transition of re-thinking a traditional medical focus care plan (described above) through to a person-centred plan, staff can initially become quite anxious, and some find it difficult to change their thinking and writing style. However, once staff have had access to a person's life story, or indeed, how they present when they have been in the care home for a few weeks, the process becomes almost second nature, and they are therefore much easier to write.

As discussed in the previous chapter, life story work is critical to planning person-centred care. As the resident living with dementia may not be able to tell us how they wish to receive their care at a given time, documented preferences when the person did have capacity or information received from relatives or friends can help us to deliver the care as closely as possible to the resident's wishes.

To demonstrate the shift between a traditional 'medical model' care plan and a person-centred care plan, the following scenario below is depicted in both the former and the latter model.

Scenario 1 (prior to life story information and person-centred training)

It has been reported by staff that 'John' has been disruptive in the dining room and keeps sliding down his chair. He pushes his food around and often needs 'feeding'. He calls out constantly and is a nuisance to the other residents in the dining room. He has lost some weight because sometimes he refuses to eat.

Example of a traditional (old culture) care plan

Need: John is disruptive at mealtimes due to his dementia

Aim: To reduce disruption and increase weight

Plan:

- Sit resident away from other residents
- Communicate to resident at all times
- Staff to feed resident to ensure he has his meals
- Staff to liaise with the GP if resident continues to be disruptive with a view to reviewing medication
- Alert GP if weight continues to decrease
- Weigh monthly
- Review care plan monthly

We note the wording in the former scenario whereby staff would use both labelling and disparaging terminology, both of which are elements of malignant social psychology and were ever present in the 'old culture of care' (Kitwood 1997).

The labels used are that John is 'disruptive' and considered a 'nuisance'. The staff are disparaging of John by laying blame on aspects of the outcomes of the mealtime experience, as if somehow this is John's fault.

The care plan itself attributes John's disruption to his dementia – a blame culture, whereby the resident (or his dementia) is at fault. Therefore, the staff do not look behind the diagnosis itself to see why John might be distressed at mealtimes, seeing the disease before the person.

Kitwood (1997) depicts the shift from old culture care to the new culture care as follows:

Person with DEMENTIA (old culture of care)

PERSON with dementia (new culture of care)

Quite simply, in the former statement, the dementia diagnosis is ever present, and the person behind the diagnosis has little significance. The illness needs managing and controlling. The second statement shows us that in the new culture of care, the person is hugely important. We need to recognise, of course, that the person has a cognitive impairment that may cause some difficulties, but if we work proactively with the person, we will reach a far greater understanding of their needs.

The aim of the care plan may not be realistic. If we are unable to address John's fundamental anxieties, then we will not increase his weight as he will still not be able to focus on a positive mealtime experience.

The plan stipulates that John should be sat away from other residents. Presumably this is so that he doesn't upset them – this step of the care plan doesn't explain why John must be sat away from other residents, immediately implying that it is for other residents' benefit rather than his own.

The next step of the plan states that the staff must communicate to the resident at all times. Again, this step doesn't tell the staff why this should be the case. Has it worked in the past? Does it reduce his anxiety or help his orientation? It would be classed as a standard phrase in a non-person-centred care plan.

The care plan then stipulates that the staff should feed John. Is this because John is unable to feed himself? Is it because staff feel that they have to because John is not eating properly and this will ensure that he gets his meal? But the staff might be disempowering John, which may, in turn, cause further frustration.

The staff then go on to consider a discussion with the GP if John continues to be disruptive, to review his medication. Note that this takes priority over the discussion with the GP to review the weight loss, as in the old culture of care – staff would generally consider this a first-line approach. The dementia is the root of the problem, the behaviour is a result of the dementia, therefore, if anti-psychotic medication is given, this would 'settle' John and the staff would be able to administer food and drink freely without disruption, and John would put on weight. In reality, however, the medication may cause further weight loss as John may become too sedated to eat properly. It may also cause him further confusion (further explained in Chapter 8).

It is then deemed that John should be weighed monthly, again a fairly standard statement, but if John is indeed losing weight, the frequency of monitoring his weight should increase to at least weekly, whereupon the GP should be contacted if staff had concerns (further explained in Chapter 5).

In summary, this care plan gives no clear direction. It is not at all person-centred and could apply to any number of residents within a care facility. It is not memorable, only as a standard script, so would staff truly understand the implications of the plan, how it applies to John as an individual, or how to deliver it?

How would staff evaluate the impact of this particular plan, as it is not particularly measurable? An increase in weight may give us an indication of whether the care plan is working, but it would be really quite difficult to evaluate most of this plan well.

Staff had also spoken to me about the difficulties they were having getting John to have a bath or a shower, and again, felt that this was because of his dementia and his confusion.

John's son was visiting the home that day so I asked if I could spend some time with him to ask him about his father, to which he gladly agreed (all names have been changed).

Scenario 2 (following conversation with John's son)

The following information was taken from my notes during an initial 20-minute conversation with John's son.

John was born in the East End of London. He came to this area when he worked in the Army carrying out his two years' National Service. He met his wife Lucy at a dance at the village hall.

John drove Heavy Goods Vehicles (HGVs) for a long time. He moved back to London and worked for the Post Office (telecommunications delivery).

John was transferred back home as Lucy's mum was poorly. His own parents died when he was 14 years old within a short space of time, and he was brought up by a neighbour, 'Aunt Izzy', who saved his life when he fell into a canal when he was nine years old. As a result of this, John has a real fear of water and will only shower – he will not go in the bath. At the seaside, John would not even go into the sea 'up to his ankles', such was his fear.

John has one son, Barry, a daughter, Carol, and another daughter, Karen (who has a learning disability).

After John's wife died (10 years ago), Karen went into a home and is now doing really well and living in a rented house with 24-hour care.

John and Lucy moved to Sunnyside Close and then four years later came to this area and lived at Larch Close. They had a lovely garden, which John took pride in. They used to have a caravan and go off for weekends before buying a static van in Bournemouth.

John was given the opportunity to become a transport manager when he was in his fifties and had to complete many qualifications and exams.

John then became Transport Manager for the Post Office Supplies Department (which later became BT Telecommunications). He has travelled all over the country.

When John 'retired' he went to work for a cider company as a night security guard. He also worked with Securicor, picking up money from the large superstores. He ended up working during the night for a large supermarket chain before finally retiring at the age of 69.

John was taking Aricept but it was upsetting his stomach, and he made a conscious decision to stop taking it.

Driving had been a large part of John's life, and the day that he received a letter from the Driver and Vehicle Licensing Agency (DVLC) to say they were taking his license away upset him deeply. He phoned his son Barry, who went over and found him on the floor having suffered a stroke.

John tried to go home after being in hospital, but this proved difficult with his mobility problems. He walked with a Zimmer frame, but had had lots of small strokes.

I asked Barry to describe John's personality:

> He is very strong willed and determined. A very loving, and caring, brilliant, father. He loved football – it was the only time he ever watched television (apart from Only Fools and Horses, which he found hilarious).
>
> Dad isn't one for mixing socially, he doesn't like being in big crowds. He was not a big drinker but if he did go to the pub he would generally just go with one person and would sit in the corner (he would never sit at the bar). He enjoys the company of two to three people and he used to like listening to what was going on around him.
>
> Dad was always absolutely immaculate; he always wore a shirt and tie and would always be coordinated.

I then asked Barry about likes and dislikes:

He loves cooked breakfasts – I think this is because he used to be on the road so much. He will eat it at any time of the day but needs the rind taken off his bacon and cutting up into small pieces now.

He doesn't like chicken at all, nor curries and stews, but likes very thinly sliced beef and ham.

He loves corned beef sandwiches and would often have a slice of corned beef, mashed potato and a fried egg (he would prefer that on Christmas day even!).

He has become very sweet toothed over the past few years and likes two to three sugars in his tea. He also likes to have tomato ketchup on all of his main meals. He would never eat a pudding before. He enjoyed an occasional lager or beer shandy.

I then asked Barry what makes John happy or sad:

Family life – he loved his family. Arguments make him really upset and he doesn't like smut or swearing. He has always been very emotional.

He would laugh at Only Fools and Horses and we have VHS videotapes at home. He also used to enjoy the Two Ronnies and Fletch. But mostly he loves music, any sort of music, and he likes listening to Radio 2 or 4.

We can immediately see that the information that John's son gave us has started to paint a very different picture, and that staff had been unwittingly working against aspects of John's life story and personality, which may ultimately have caused his distress.

John's son was glad to help, although initially he was quite surprised that things from John's distant past might affect his current frame of mind and well-being. The short time spent with Barry enabled us to formulate many new care plans relating to increasing his well-being, helping him with his personal hygiene needs and tailoring his activity preference.

I spoke to John's named nurse and his key worker after I had spoken to Barry, and shared the information that we had gained. The information generated a lot of discussion amongst us as to how the information we now had could explain some of the aspects of care that John was not happy with, namely, his 'refusal' to bathe or shower and the 'disruption' at mealtimes. It was quite clear that John needed his individual choices to be recognised, his personality to be taken into account and his past fears to be both acknowledged and validated.

As a group, we sat and discussed person-centred approaches and developed two new care plans for John.

Example of a person-centred care plan

Need: John has lost six kg in weight over the past two months

Aim: To help John to enjoy his meals and increase his weight

Plan:

- John likes to have tomato ketchup on all his savoury meals
- John needs some assistance to cut up his food
- John dislikes stews, casseroles, curries, and chicken
- John likes corned beef hash, sliced beef and ham and corned beef sandwiches
- John loves his puddings and should be offered another pudding if he does not eat his dinner
- John likes two to three sugars in his tea
- John enjoys an occasional beer or lager shandy
- John doesn't like big crowds so would not enjoy going into the dining room but may prefer to sit with one or two people in a smaller room, or perhaps his own room
- John likes a cooked breakfast and will eat it at any time of the day

- John might wake in the night for something to eat as he used to work nights as a security guard
- Provide a snack box for John to enable him to freely access nutritional snacks
- Weigh John weekly (and complete nutritional assessment)
- Discuss with GP if John continues to lose weight
- Communicate new care plan to all staff
- Evaluate care plan weekly initially until John's weight has improved

This person-centred care plan demonstrates John's uniqueness. It could not be applied to any other person because it is so specific to John's individual needs, preferences and choices.

This person-centred plan is also easier to remember. When we tried this out at a teaching session, although the former more traditional care plan was much shorter, staff could not recall any specifics, but gleefully shouted out all of the aspects of the second care plan, because they had remembered the detail.

When the care plan was shared with the staff team at handovers, staff suggested that a conservatory that was not used on a regular basis could form a new small dining area that could be used for John and a couple of other residents who he seemed to get along with.

The chef was also informed of John's new plan; he needed to get lots of corned beef in! The staff were quite disbelieving at first of step 1, and thought it quite strange that John would want tomato ketchup on a roast beef dinner. John, however, was delighted, and ate all of his meals. He quickly became semi-independent again and his weight increased. Mealtimes were no longer a battle for John or the staff, and John once again began to look forward to his meals.

Second example of a person-centred care plan

Need: John can occasionally become tearful and anxious

Aim: To maintain John's psychological well-being

Plan:

- Maintain John's individual needs, and particularly his dressing preferences, as John always like to be very smart
- John has a real fear of water, does not like to go into the bath and has always taken a shower
- John doesn't like to be in a crowd, so perhaps he could have his lunch or tea in a smaller area, with one or two people
- John likes to listen to his music, so staff need to put on a CD or turn the radio on to Radio 2 or 4
- John likes to watch Only Fools and Horses or football on the television on occasions
- John adores his family and we need to facilitate contact with his son and daughters
- Pictures of John's family to be placed on the wall or in an album
- If John's dietary needs are not met, John can become upset, so please follow his dietary plan (attached)
- John might feel trapped at times as he used to travel all over the country and he loved to go in his garden, so we need to encourage John to go out when he can with either a member of staff or his family
- Holiday photos of caravan weekends and holidays to be put in an album for John to look at
- Encourage John to express his emotions and support him whilst he relates his fears and anxieties or memories
- Try and encourage John to join in with some activities in a small group, perhaps darts, dominoes or cards. We might be able to involve John in the gardening.

- Arrange for a daily newspaper to come into the home so that John can read it
- Ask John if he would like to go to his room if any of the other residents are getting upset (as John gets distressed by arguments and/or swearing)

These two care plan examples demonstrate how different the traditional care plan versus the person-centred care plan can be. The very simple step of introducing the resident's name immediately brings the resident into focus, and enables staff to remember that they are developing care interventions in partnership with the resident themselves.

A person is a person through others. (Bryden 2005, p127)

Chapter 5

Getting the 'Fundamentals' Right

Sue Goldsmith

In this chapter, I focus on the importance of getting the 'fundamentals' of care right, and explain what the fundamental care aspects are. If we are applying a person-centred approach, we need to take a holistic view of the person's needs in order to optimise their opportunity for well-being.

What exactly are fundamental care needs? The government has recently announced that all care staff should be trained in fundamental needs (DH 2013), and deem this to include helping people to eat and wash and to be helped to turn in bed to prevent pressure sores – in essence, essential physical health care needs.

Some would argue that psychological, spiritual and sociological needs are equally as fundamental as physical needs. For the most part I would agree, but we need to ensure that the essential physical needs of someone living with dementia are met before we can hope to achieve any of the other needs successfully.

Maslow described a hierarchy of basic human needs (Figure 5.1), and Poston summarises how Level 1, physiological needs, were initially established when Maslow, following an observation of monkeys, noted that given the choice between food and play or water and play, the monkeys would always choose either food and/or water (Poston 2009).

Later on in his work, Maslow transferred his findings to human beings, and noted that each level of the pyramid he depicted needed to be met before people could progress up it to what he termed 'self-actualisation'. In terms of providing fundamental or essential care needs within a care home environment, I refer to Level 1, physiological care needs. The chapters within this book that focus on life story, activity and reducing distress all contribute to helping the resident to achieve Levels 2, 3 and 4.

By applying all that we know that is written within the text of this book, we should be able to reach the very top level of self-actualisation (Level 5), where a resident is deemed to be reaching their full potential.

RESPECTING RESIDENTS

It goes without saying that all of the following guidance should be carried out with the utmost respect for the residents in our care. Would any of us wish for somebody else to be carrying out our personal care, to view and cleanse intimate parts of our bodies? Residents are bound to feel both embarrassed and guilty that this needs to be done for them, and our job is to ensure that we try to reduce their embarrassment as much as we can, and to relieve them of any guilt they might feel through sensitive approaches and communication.

Of course, we should always encourage and facilitate residents to do as much as they are able, as this will both foster their level of independence and reduce any feelings of guilt or embarrassment.

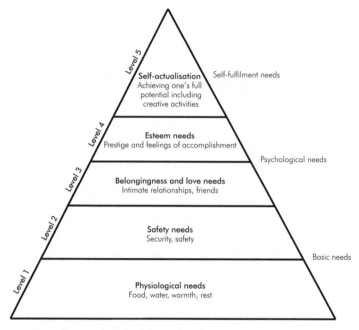

Figure 5.1: Diagram of Maslow's hierarchy of needs

TIME TO CARE

Commissioners of care really need to ensure that additional time is factored in when providing personal care for somebody living with dementia. In a world that can seem extremely confusing and unreal, any attempt to rush somebody with a cognitive impairment is bound to result in increased distress for both the person being cared for and the person attempting to administer the care.

Each approach and intervention needs to be explained using both verbal and non-verbal language. The person being cared for needs time to receive, retain and process the information being given to them and time to formulate a response. This is fairly immediate for those of who are fortunate enough to have full cognition, but for a person living with dementia, they may need additional time to respond.

HELPING RESIDENTS TO EAT AND DRINK WELL

This particular element of fundamental care is covered in depth in Chapter 6 in relation to making mealtime an activity and a focus. For this chapter, we need to look at what we consider to be the very essence of helping a resident to eat and drink well.

Our first priority is to establish the resident's choice of food. What do they like, and perhaps more importantly, what don't they like? An uninformed carer may dismiss an uneaten meal as a sign that the resident is not hungry. The resident themself may not be able to articulate that they do not like the food, and simply push it around their plate or spit it out, even though they are extremely hungry. I would do the same with a corned beef hash!

If a resident is partial to a particular food, it can be extremely helpful to offer this more often if they are not eating particularly well for a period of time. Nutritionists may scold me severely, but if a resident is not eating well but would eat two portions of their favourite pudding (providing they are not diabetic), what harm can there be, particularly if the person is nearing the end of their life?

Residents need to be supported physically to eat and drink well – comfortable positioning, either in the chair or in the bed, close to a table and with the appropriate 'tools for the job'. There are many adaptations that can be used to assist a person to eat well:

- 'sticky mats' to stop the plate or bowl sliding
- coloured crockery to provide a better contrast
- moulded cutlery to help to provide a better grip
- lipped plates and bowls

- two-handled mugs
- mugs with lids and a spout.

Time is also a really important factor here. Residents may take longer to eat a meal, and this doesn't necessarily mean that they do not want it or are not enjoying it. Smaller portions could be presented so that the meal does not go cold as quickly, with a further portion being offered once the first portion is consumed (see Chapter 6).

Staff also need to consider mouth care of the resident and their ability to chew – are their dentures fitting well? Are they having problems with their own teeth? Does the resident have any mouth ulcers or oral thrush? Is the resident able to swallow properly, or do they need a referral to a speech and language therapist via the resident's GP?

It is difficult to function if we are hungry or thirsty, and if a resident is not able to express their need or has difficulties that we are not able to resolve, this could lead to serious malnutrition or dehydration. We have found that generally it is not an outcome of the diagnosis of dementia that the resident will lose weight, as many of our residents have actually increased their weight.

HELPING RESIDENTS TO TAKE CARE OF THEIR SKIN

As with food and drink, we only have to think of ourselves when trying to determine what a resident in our care may need if they are not fully able to articulate or carry out their care independently.

Within the care homes, staff will complete a skin assessment, which helps to highlight if the resident is at particular risk of their skin breaking down, which in turn helps us to implement additional prevention strategies such as air mattresses, air cushions or repositioning regimes.

But back to the obvious – a resident with dry skin will need regular moisturising or it may become itchy and sore. A resident who does not remain continent will need help to cleanse and dry the skin as soon as possible so that the urine does not burn the skin (although the newer continence aids do keep urine away from the skin).

If a resident has a pressure ulcer, they may need regular pain relief, particularly prior to the dressing taking place, to minimise any pain that may be experienced during the dressing change.

HELPING RESIDENTS TO MEET THEIR NEED FOR THE TOILET

It is helpful for staff to carry out at least a week of monitoring when the resident is first admitted to the care home to establish what might be their usual toilet routine. As human beings, we are all very different, and our continence patterns will vary enormously.

If we can establish a 'usual' time that a resident is likely to either pass urine or open their bowels, we can ensure going forward that we encourage the resident to visit the toilet prior to the times we have documented, to try and maintain continence.

As the resident's cognitive ability declines, staff should also look for non-verbal and verbal signs that the resident may want to use the toilet. For some this may be starting to 'fiddle' with their zip. For others, this may manifest in the resident calling out, but not necessarily asking for the toilet, as they are unable to find the words.

As with other areas of personal care, staff should ensure that they offer the resident the upmost dignity and empower them to be as independent as possible.

HELPING RESIDENTS TO GET WASHED AND DRESSED

Most of us take a shower or a bath daily, but we should not place our own expectations on others. When I think of my own grandparents, in their later years, they found it really difficult to get into the bath and would have what they called a 'strip wash' at the sink. My gramp would have a shave everyday (as does my father), but my husband shaves every two to three days as his skin becomes sore. There is almost an expectation that we should deliver these things every day to keep people 'looking nice', but are they feeling nice? Prior to admission and during the first days of the resident coming into the home, we should work with the resident and their family to establish a preferred routine, and this should then be documented in the resident's care plan so that all staff can use the same approach.

Establishing the resident's choice is so important. It can be a critical point regarding the preference for a bath, shower or strip wash, as any offering that deviates away from the resident's preference may potentially lead to distress, as it would move away from what they were used to.

Receiving help to get washed and dressed in a dignified manner is also a fundamental right of each person. We should recognise that, like us, the resident has done this for themself up until this point and again, like us, may find it embarrassing and humiliating to now need assistance. Recognising this allows us first to ensure that we are sensitive in our approach and that we have started to establish a relationship with the resident by spending some time with them. Imagine how it might feel to be assisted with washing or bathing by someone you don't know, like or trust? We also need to make sure that we have taken every measure to maintain the person's dignity. I used to look after a lady who would only be assisted 'in two halves' and who used to become inconsolable if she was ever asked to take all of her clothes off at once. We used towels and loose fitting shirts to help her to feel safe and to maintain her dignity; she even bathed in a shirt and used to enjoy a bath in this way more than anybody I have ever cared for since!

The bathing environment within a care home can often be the place where residents living with dementia may feel most vulnerable; this is where the most intimate care is likely to take place and the resident may very well feel at a disadvantage as they are partially clothed and requiring sensitive assistance. It is vital that staff recognise just how vulnerable the resident may feel, and try to view the experience from the resident's perspective.

The physical environment of the bathroom, often quite clinical and with intimidating hoisting equipment, can be a contributing factor to this apprehension and distress, and it is important to try to create a more homely, less clinical feel to the bathing environment. A warm, relaxing room with similar pictures and bathroom accessories to those you would have in your own home can help to orientate the resident to the purpose of being in the room. This, combined with affording residents time and encouraging them to be active in their own care, will allow them to remain in control of the situation – a key element in maintaining high levels of self-esteem and minimising feelings of distress.

HELPING RESIDENTS TO MAINTAIN GOOD MOUTH CARE

A focus on mouth care is also a necessity of meeting fundamental care needs, and it is important to gain an insight into the oral health of the resident on admission. An assessment of the health status of the mouth, lips, natural teeth and/or dentures will help staff to establish the type of oral health support required, and ensure that this care is planned for.

Recent studies of older people have indicated that a third of the people surveyed experience dental pain or discomfort, and over half regularly or always experience difficulty in choosing appropriate food, experience speech difficulties and feel conscious of their general appearance (Gluzman *et al.* 2012). For residents living with dementia, they may not always be able to tell staff that they are experiencing discomfort or pain. Staff need to be proactive when promoting oral health, and ensure it is given equal priority to other elements of fundamental care by enabling regular dental check-ups and ensuring daily oral care. The simple act of regularly assisting a resident to clean natural teeth or thoroughly clean dentures can reduce the risk of aspiration pneumonia and chronic oral thrush. Staff should also look for signs of oral ill health such as a decrease in appetite, a change in behaviour that may be caused by pain or discomfort, reluctance to speak or inability to tolerate drinks of a certain temperature. Early identification and treatment of oral problems can prevent unnecessary suffering and feelings of ill-being.

HELPING RESIDENTS TO LOOK AFTER THEIR FEET

Equal importance should be given to foot care and the impact that this can have on residents when this is not maintained. Imagine not being able to walk anymore because your toenails are too long and your shoes no longer fit or because you experience painful bunions. Imagine the feelings of frustration, anger and vulnerability as your independence is stripped away from you. A resident who may not be able to verbalise the reasons for their distress may demonstrate this in other ways; therefore it is important that staff assess and monitor the health of residents' feet on a regular basis.

On admission staff should visually assess residents' feet and take into account the health of the skin, any sore areas, bunions, corns and state of their toe nails. Any observations should prompt discussion with the resident and their family regarding how these issues have been treated and, where possible, a continuation of this treatment by the same practitioners should be sought. Daily foot care to prevent worsening of existing conditions or to maintain healthy feet should be included in the care plan, and staff should aim to keep feet clean and dry at all times.

HELPING RESIDENTS TO DRESS IN CLOTHING OF THEIR CHOICE

Every person is unique and has an individual sense of style and preference when it comes to how they dress and the way they choose to look. For some of us it would be unthinkable to leave the house without first applying our make-up or combing our hair. Maintaining our appearance can be an indicator of well-being, and we also need to recognise that this is also the case for residents living with dementia (Well-being Profiling Tool, Bradford Dementia Group discussed further on page 177).

Historically, care has sometimes been given that has been in the interests of staff rather than the person receiving care. This has included the selection of clothing with the view that it is 'easier' to assist a person who is wearing loose clothing such as sweatshirts and tracksuit bottoms. As a person who has never owned a pair of tracksuit bottoms, I would find it incredibly confusing to suddenly be dressed in these because it was easier for somebody else. Not only would I try to remove them, it would also have an impact on my well-being and my sense of identity.

Enabling residents to continue to choose their own clothing is a simple step in helping them to maintain control over their lives and to maintain identity. During the pre-admission process it is useful to document these choices and also to identify the method that a resident will use to choose their own clothing. Too often I have read that someone is no longer able to choose what they wish to wear, and in the next entry the staff member is describing how the resident is 'stripping off' in the lounge! It is important that we start to look at the non-verbal signs that may indicate to us the choices and preferences that individual residents are still able to make. Some residents continue to be able to choose by saying what they wish to wear; others may need to see the clothes in order to be able to choose. Ensuring that a resident's personal preferences are respected can be the difference between well-being and ill-being. Simple choices such as slippers or shoes, bra or vest, nightdress or pyjamas all contribute to an overall feeling of being empowered and in control of our lives.

HELPING RESIDENTS TO FEEL COMFORTABLE

Physical comfort is a basic human need and is essential to ensuring that every person has a basis for well-being. Care home chairs, however expensive and inviting they appear, can become uncomfortable after a time. I always try to liken this to long journeys that I have experienced, either by train or plane, and remember how irritable and frustrated I became by having limited or restricted movement. I inevitably cause much annoyance to travelling companions as I cross and uncross my legs in a bid to get comfortable or shift around in my seat searching for the most padded part of my backside to rest on. I may then spend a few minutes slumped in a very poor position while I read a magazine or book and then moan (and possibly even swear!) when my back is aching. I don't want to talk to anyone, eat anything and I feel utterly miserable. Now imagine that this is a resident in your care, but added to this, the resident is unable to move independently, and therefore can't cross and uncross legs in a bid to get comfortable or shift around in their seat. In addition to this, they no longer have the verbal ability to say 'I'm not comfortable'. This physical discomfort may well set the scene for how they feel for the rest of the day and have an impact on their desire to eat, engage and generally participate in everyday life. As discussed in other chapters, the effects of ill-being, depression and poor appetite can quickly lead to other physical and psychological health needs – ensuring that residents' basic comfort needs are met can go a long way to forming a positive basis for well-being.

So is it enough to ensure a resident in your care is washed, dressed and assisted to a chair before moving on to the next task? The key to any care practice is to move away from task-orientated thinking and instead ask, 'What does the person want?' That thought has become the vein of person-centred care, and throughout the programme we always prompt staff to remind themselves of this, to constantly observe and to ask, and to accept that decisions are not set in stone, and that as fickle human beings we have the right and the mind set to change our decisions at any time!

Preparing the basics to promote comfort is our starting point. Ensuring we have good knowledge with regard to the individual is vital – what pre-existing conditions may cause them pain or discomfort? A resident who has chronic arthritis and now also has a diagnosis of dementia still has arthritis! Therefore we have to ensure that we don't 'forget' this, as physical health is also a contributory factor in a person's experience of their dementia journey (Kitwood 1997). The importance of effective pain relief and the monitoring of this is explored further in Chapter 11, and is something that should be in the forefront of each care worker's mind when caring for people living with dementia. We also need to be aware of the risk of skin breakdown, and the correct use of an appropriate risk assessment tool (Waterlow or Braden) can help staff to identify any risks and put measures into place to reduce these. Knowing whether residents are able to reposition themselves independently is also vital, as it will play a major part in the planning of individualised care regarding pressure relief. This will include whether there is a need for specific pressure-relieving equipment such as a cushion or mattress, and how often the resident will need help to reposition. If a resident also spends long periods sitting, it is important to check that the chair is the right chair, whether it is ergonomically suited to the person, and whether it has the right pressure-relieving properties. Occupational therapists have excellent knowledge in this area and are quite happy to advise.

Temperature is another area of basic comfort need. I am a person who always feels the cold regardless of season, and it is rare that I am seen in short sleeves. My colleagues regularly hear me complaining about how cold it is, and I am quick to move if a window is opened during a meeting; I have even been known to sit in jeans and a coat on a foreign beach! This is unlikely to change for me as I get older, and I can't envisage my future without my trusted cardigans and dressing gowns. So how might I feel if I lived in a care home and the staff didn't know this about me? If, because they were warm from rushing about, they assumed I was warm enough too? I would be miserable, angry that they hadn't noticed I was cold, and would not be able to focus on what I was supposed to be doing or what was going on around me. If I was no longer able to find the right words to tell staff that I was cold, then my anger and frustration would no doubt increase and manifest in my actions; would I then be labelled as having 'challenging behaviour'? Knowing your resident, being mindful of room temperature and open windows and looking for clues (both verbal and non-verbal) are all simple measures we can take that don't take any extra time but can, for the individual, be the difference between well-being and ill-being.

HELPING RESIDENTS TO SLEEP WELL

Refreshing sleep is vital to well-being, and sleep deprivation during the night may lead to increased sleepiness during the day and reduced cognitive functioning (Neubauer 1999). Therefore helping residents to sleep well is an important factor in optimising well-being, and there are several elements to this that proactive practitioners should be aware of and should be striving to meet. We all have different routines and a preference regarding our sleep pattern, and it is important that staff try their best to adhere to these routines. Historically, in care home settings, the routines that have been established have been to suit the needs of the staff rather than the residents being cared for. As a night nurse for many years, I am saddened to say that at times in the past I would focus on the needs of my staff rather than the residents. I would moan that so few people were in bed when I started my shift without thinking about what each resident preferred to do, and going to work became quite a negative experience. After a few months of feeling this way, 'the penny dropped' and I came to the realisation that my colleagues on the day shift weren't lazy, as I had initially thought, but instead far more person-centred than I was. By changing my thinking and going with what each resident wanted rather than what I wanted, working during the evening and the night became an opportunity to get to know each resident as a person, and to share their joys, fears, laughter and tears. As a result, residents slept better, experienced less distress, and had the opportunity to enjoy some much needed 'chill out' time at a time of day that was quieter and more relaxed.

So how can we achieve this? The starting point for this is to establish what the resident's individual sleep needs are, and what their routine is. As mentioned before, we all have different routines and this is no different for our residents! I like to change into my pyjamas and dressing gown straight after my evening meal; I then like to watch television with a glass (or two) of vodka and diet coke. This is my chill out time and I am relaxed and ready for bed by 10pm. My husband, on the other hand, does not own a pair of pyjamas or dressing gown; he changes into a clean T-shirt and tracksuit bottoms after having a shower straight after tea. He then likes to potter around the house and the garage until well after midnight, when he will come to bed. Could we fit into a care home environment? Probably not. Could a care home environment fit around our routines? Most definitely! If the staff took the time to get to know us and strive to give us what we want and are used to, then there should be no reason why we wouldn't sleep well in a care home environment.

Other equally simple considerations can also contribute to our residents sleeping well. Ensuring that residents have a full and stimulating day can reduce daytime napping caused by boredom. Being involved in meaningful activities and the day-to-day running of the home can mean that residents are ready to sleep during the night, and this may help to reduce periods of waking at night.

Ensuring that residents are physically warm and comfortable during the night can also help with sleep. This also includes making sure that any pain relief that is needed is offered. Ensuring that residents are not hungry or thirsty before they go to bed and that they are offered a snack and a drink if they awaken during the night is also important.

Encouraging residents and their families to make bedrooms more personalised and therefore appearing more familiar can also promote a conducive environment for sleep. Familiar bedding or a special pillow can be the difference between a good and a bad night's sleep.

Staff also need to consider possible psychological barriers to sleep. Is the resident frightened of being on their own? Are they used to sleeping in a single bed? Are they startled by the unfamiliar sounds in a strange environment? These are all questions that care staff should ask if someone is experiencing disturbed sleep. Monitoring sleep patterns over a 24-hour period is also good practice when trying to help a resident to achieve restful sleep. Napping during the day may lead to sleepless nights, so it is important that this information is captured.

Night sedation should not be seen as the norm for residents in our care homes. An important element of the PEARL (Positively Enriching And enhancing Residents' Lives) programme has been to look at promoting person-centred care over a 24-hour period. Recognising that what we do in the day influences how we sleep at night has had a major impact in reducing the prescription of hypnotic medication for our residents. In addition, the implementation of measures to ensure all fundamental care needs are met can also lead to improved sleeping experiences and an overall increased quality of life.

As discussed throughout this chapter, getting the fundamentals right is key to quality care. The fundamentals are the foundations, the basis on which excellent specialised dementia care can be built. We can all do this, but the most important factor is *how* we do this in order that the resident perceives it as good quality care. The PEARL programme is about recognising that the 'how' needs to be adapted for each individual resident, and is a tool that allows that culture change to occur; in turn, this returns the focus of care to the person rather than the service providing the care. Providing all of the fundamentals requires the ability of all staff to be able to communicate effectively, to be able to recognise and respond to the communication style of each resident in order to find out what care they want to receive. By looking for non-verbal clues as well as listening to the spoken word we are truly starting to hear what our residents are trying to tell us. By waiting for opportunities rather than imposing task-focused routines we are allowing residents to maintain control over their lives; and by looking for the meaning behind actions and words, we are truly striving to understand life from the resident's perspective.

Chapter 6

Making the Most of Mealtimes

Jason Corrigan

In this chapter, I look at the mealtime experience within the care home, and describe how we have implemented research and evidence-based practice to improve nutrition, and ultimately helped our residents to gain weight. Most of us enjoy our meals and especially look forward to dining out, and this should not be any different for a person living with dementia in a care home. Historically, it has been a given that people with a diagnosis of dementia will lose weight because of their condition. However, under the PEARL (Positively Enriching And enhancing Residents' Lives) programme the vast majority of residents actually increase their weight. But how can this be achieved?

I would like to start this chapter by providing you with two scenarios around possible experiences of eating.

Scenario 1

You arrive at a restaurant and are asked what table you would like to sit at; you make your decision and the person walks you to the table and pulls the chair out so that you can sit down. The table is set in a welcoming manner with a tablecloth, cutlery, napkin, condiments, table arrangement, and you feel warm and in a relaxed state. You are asked if you would like a drink, and you choose what you would like. You are then handed a menu to assist you in choosing your meal. The menu provides a full description of what meals are available, and you take your time in deliberating what it is you would like.

You place your order and enjoy your drink, and start a conversation with your companion and await your meal. There is soft background music playing and this adds to a relaxed atmosphere.

Your meal arrives and it looks very appetising, and you sit and enjoy you meal at your pace. You're already looking forward to seeing the dessert menu as you know that is going to taste just as good.

When you leave the restaurant you feel content and happy and you just know you will return.

Scenario 2

You arrive at the same restaurant the following day and you are welcomed through the door. You are not asked were you would like to sit, but are shown to a table where there are already people sat. Some of the people look familiar, but you don't really know them.

The table is not set, apart from a knife and a fork that are placed in front of you. You are poured a drink of tea from a big teapot that you notice is being taken around all of the other tables.

The restaurant seems rather noisy with the staff chatting amongst themselves, rushing around from table to table, occasionally glancing over at you and smiling. You begin to feel somewhat uncomfortable as no one sat at the table is talking, so you stand up to leave. One of the staff comes over and asks you to sit down as your meal is nearly ready.

At that point you are approached from behind and a 'bib' type apron is put around your neck. It covers most of your clothes and one of the staff says to you, 'Just in case you spill'. Though you'd like to think that their intentions are well meant, you feel embarrassed, child-like and wonder how the others sat at the table may view you.

At that point your meal arrives, and though it does look appetising, you can't help but wonder who ordered this meal for you, and also why your dessert has been put on the table at the same time.

You eat your meal in a hurried manner as you don't want to let your dessert go cold, and you also want to go and sit back in the comfy armchair that you had not long left behind.

You leave the restaurant and feel relieved to be away from the environment and all the hustle and bustle, hoping you do not have to return, or if you do, that it will be a better experience.

As you can see, two quite different scenarios; however, both are based on true accounts. The first scenario and experience was my own, as a customer recently in a local restaurant, going out for a meal with a friend. Sadly and shamefully the second scenario (which was a regular occurrence) was that of myself as a carer, assisting at mealtimes back in the 1980s when I was working in a local care home, and the experiences I describe, well, I often reflect and wonder if that's how my actions made the residents feel at the time, and why my personal experience was not reflected within my work place at the time?

EXCUSE OR REALITY?

I struggle now to come to terms with the reasons staff members sometimes give for not being able to provide a pleasant, person-centred approach to mealtimes. Having worked in the care sector for 26 years I have seen and been a part of both task-orientated teams and also teams that deliver truly person-centred care. If one home is able to achieve the latter, then why can't others? After all, being person-centred is about values and approaches not degrees and diplomas. Sabat (2010) states, 'people with dementia are affected by the ways they are treated by healthy others in social situations. They can retain aspects of selfhood including self-personae, but the latter depends on how they are treated by others' (p.82), and certainly my experiences appear to echo this.

Mealtimes in the care home can be one of the busiest periods of the day, and staff often don't realise the importance of providing a relaxed and calm mealtime experience for those people living with dementia, as they often rush around trying to get the 'task' completed by a set time, and from my many experiences and observations, usually to appease other members of the staff team. Brooker (2010) tells us that, 'When people are very dependent on care services, quality of life becomes inextricably linked with quality of care' (p.476), and it is therefore crucial that the quality that is provided is truly person-centred, and by founding and maintaining relationships, this enables carers to promote identity, personhood and ensure that when needs change, then so does the service provision.

Nutritional intake is clearly part of providing fundamental care. However, when intake decreases, the reasons behind this are often overlooked without consideration being given not only to the consequences of regular poor dietary intake, but also to possible causes or events that can also have an impact and determine if someone has had a pleasurable experience at mealtimes or not; this is when the biomedical approach is usually taken. Kitwood (1997) refers to this approach as 'neuropathic ideology' where the dementia as an illness is given solely as the reason for any change within the person.

From food presentation to nutritional values, the dining environment to celebrations and cultural beliefs, mealtimes are an essential element to any person's day and can also impact on a person's well-being and their physical health. Therefore, as a company, we take seriously the importance of making the most of mealtimes to ensure it is a pleasant and enjoyable experience for everyone.

At the very heart of the programme is an holistic approach that engages all key influencers of a resident living with dementia care experiences, including relatives, friends, staff, community clinicians and general practitioners (GPs), to help focus on the individualisation of each resident living with dementia. With this approach, elements of the programme focus on nutrition and the mealtime experience to ensure that a truly person-centred approach is embedded into the culture of the home, and this is also supported by a dedicated information section on nutrition and mealtimes for all staff to undertake as part of their training, so they are fully aware of the many factors that incorporate making the most of mealtimes. To further enhance staff knowledge as a company, we have devised a quality dining audit that ensures the staff review, monitor and adapt the mealtime experience. The audit comprises of 65 questions, broken down into five sections that different staff will monitor during a mealtime experience, recording their experience and feedback to the remainder of the staff. The audit is carried out once every six months.

Every one of us, regardless of any illness or disability, should be afforded an enjoyable dining experience, and just because you may live in a care home, this should be no different. Of course there may have to be adjustments made to compensate for how dementia may be impacting on an individual to ensure all needs are being met; however, does that not come under one's duty of care?

THE INCLUSIVE ENVIRONMENT

An inclusive environment is essential, and starts with appropriate signage to ensure residents are able to locate the dining area within a home. Signage with both pictures and words is a very good way of ensuring that residents living with dementia can identify what the main purpose of each room is.

During mealtimes, staff should ensure that noise levels are minimal within the dining area (for example, the noise of banging crockery, staff conversations with each other, staff shouting out to each other, should all be avoided). Staff may also want to consider playing 'gentle' music within the dining room to help provide a relaxed atmosphere; however, any music that is played should be the residents' choice or of a suitable genre.

Protected mealtimes plays a fundamental part in ensuring that residents are not unnecessarily distracted from eating their meals, and therefore the staff team must recognise that mealtimes are an important part of the day for residents living with dementia, and may indeed become a focused activity. Therefore, medication (unless prescribed to be taken with food) should not be administered during mealtimes as this may distract residents or discourage them from eating any more as it may have tainted their taste palate. Relatives should also (but sensitively) be discouraged from visiting at mealtimes unless they like to assist their loved ones in eating their food, and if this is the case, then this should be encouraged and facilitated. Staff must also ensure that any visits to the home by others are not arranged at mealtimes including GPs, district nurses etc., as breaking a resident's concentration may result in them not continuing with their meal – none of us should be disturbed when we are eating and enjoying our food.

There is no reason whatsoever that tables cannot be set with tablecloths, place mats, crockery, cutlery, condiments etc. within a dementia care setting, despite numerous excuses often given for the reasons they are not. I have often heard staff say we can't put flowers on the table as they may get eaten; they cannot put a tablecloth on as it may get pulled off, etc. My advice would be to look at the possible reasons behind these events. If staff did observe a resident attempting to eat flowers, then perhaps the resident may be hungry and therefore food could be offered as an alternative. Perhaps some residents may want to be involved in the setting of tables or clearing away and feel they just want to help? Consideration also needs to be given how far in advance tables are set for meals, as this may cause added confusion for some people who may think that the meal is about to be served when in fact it is not.

When laying tables for mealtimes, staff also need to ensure that appropriate colour contrast is used to aid residents to easily identify items. For example, you would not place white crockery on a white tablecloth, as those residents with visual impairment would then find it hard to distinguish.

Tables and chairs also need careful consideration to ensure they are comfortable and practicable. For example, can a dining chair be pushed up close to a table to help a person to reach their meal, or does the design of the chair or height of the table prevent this?

For those residents whose mobility is poor and who require assistance into the dining room, staff need to consider the dignity and level of comfort that leaving a resident in the wheelchair to eat their meal has, and any decision that is made must be in the best interest of the resident and not what is easiest for the staff team.

When looking at the dining environment, staff also need to consider that some residents may prefer to eat their meals in another part of the home, for example, their bedroom or the lounge, though as mentioned above, this must be the choice of the resident, and any 'tray' service should be set to the same standard as the dining table.

I have often come across residents having their meal in the lounge area sat in a chair with their meal placed on a cantilever table, and it has been left to go cold. Communication is essential at mealtimes, whether it is to offer gentle prompts or to promote a sense of belonging, and therefore staff need to appreciate that mealtimes cannot be a hurried experience, including for those residents who need assistance to eat their meals.

On a similar note, staff need to ensure that all residents who choose to do so are afforded the opportunity to have their meal in the dining area, and therefore consideration needs to be given to the size of the dining room to ensure it does not become overcrowded. This may require the staff team to look at introducing two sittings for mealtimes or staggered mealtimes. Where this has happened within our care homes it has had a positive impact, not only for the residents, but also for staff who have commented on how much more relaxed they have found the experience, and that they have more time to spend with the residents.

Many of our care homes are now providing the main meal of the day in the early evening and moving away from serving this at the traditional lunchtime period. The rationale behind this is that most homes provide a staggered cooked breakfast, and therefore by midday, most residents were either not hungry or only eating small amounts of food.

Where this is now practised, homes have reported better nutritional intake for residents, better sleeping patterns for residents and less food wastage then was previously the case.

ENABLING CHOICE

Good practice would be for staff to attempt to establish likes and dislikes, portion sizes and food preferences prior to or on the day of admission of a resident to the care home, and to pass this information to both the catering team and all other staff working within the home. If the resident is unable to communicate their wishes (pictorial prompts could be used), staff should then contact relatives or family to ascertain this information.

If residents do not have any family, staff will need to establish likes and dislikes by a process of elimination, by sensitively observing and recording their findings within relevant care documentation so that the resident's preferences can be shared amongst the staff, including the catering team (this also includes sharing information in relation to any special dietary requirements or any changes in dietary requirements).

Menu choices should be offered on the day, rather than the day before, as for some residents living with dementia, they may find it difficult to retain the information they provided previously. When staff are providing meals for residents (who have not been able to vocalise their choice), staff should present both choices (plated) to the person to enable them to point to the meal that they would like, and be mindful that some residents may change their mind. A good example of this was a resident living in a care home who happened to point to both dishes being shown to them. The staff obliged and the resident ate both meals.

When choices are made for mealtimes each course, when served, must be served individually after the resident has finished with their previous course. For example, desserts should not be put in front of a resident whilst they are still eating their main meal or left on a trolley somewhere going cold. We only have to think how we would feel if this happened to us whilst eating in a restaurant.

Staff also need to take into account that although the care documentation may indicate likes and dislikes, people's tastes and preferences may change, and therefore residents must always be offered choices on a daily basis. For example, I may prefer to drink coffee most days, but I do occasionally like a cup of tea depending on my mood at the time.

The catering team in any home provides a vital service, and good practice would suggest that they introduce themselves to the residents soon after admission, and regularly seek feedback from residents and their relatives on the quality of food served.

FACILITATING INDEPENDENCE

Care homes should be about facilitating independence and promoting strengths rather than de-skilling residents. This is often not done with bad intent but is often more to do with saving time to ensure the shift runs like clockwork. Staff need to appreciate and realise that when working in any job where you are providing a care service for another human being, no two days will ever be the same, and time cannot be seen as the factor of a successful day.

Time is a really important factor, however, when it comes to mealtimes, as some residents may take longer to eat a meal; this doesn't necessarily mean that they do not want it or are not enjoying it. Smaller portions could be presented so that the meal does not go cold as quickly, with a further portion being offered once the first portion is consumed. The pace of mealtimes, wherever they take place, should be set by the residents, and adequate staffing levels need to be taken into account at these times.

When assistance is afforded to residents who are deemed to require assistance, we should be careful not to disempower those who do not need help, even though it would be easier or quicker for staff if they did receive it – for example, a resident is taking a long time to eat their meal and so staff assist them, or a resident who begins to eat their meal with their fingers is discouraged from doing so. For those residents who require assistance, staff should always sit with them, maintaining eye contact and communicating intermittently without overpowering them.

Prompts may be needed if the resident is unable to recognise the meal, and staff should seek clarification of enjoyment of the meal through either verbal or non-verbal observations. All food should be offered to residents in a dignified manner and at a pace that is acceptable to the resident, and if the staff are also able to eat at the same time as residents, this further adds to a sense of inclusiveness and relationship building.

Staff should ascertain whether residents need any adaptations to assist them to eat independently (for example, adapted cutlery or crockery), and where this has been identified, then we must ensure it is provided to promote independence. I recall as a home manager trying for many months to get staff to see that that removing a person's independence is morally wrong and not the role of a care home.

Staff must also recognise that residents with dementia may not always select the appropriate cutlery to eat their meal (for example, a spoon rather than a fork, fingers rather than cutlery). However, it must be recognised that this is the resident's choice and it is helping to maintain their independence, and sometimes, by replacing the cutlery, the resident may feel disempowered or ridiculed (disparaged) and stop eating. When dealing with situations like this staff must use their judgement (and their knowledge and relationship with the resident) as to how the resident is likely to respond to any sensitive intervention.

Staff may also observe that if it is a continuous approach by a resident to attempt to eat their meal with their fingers, they should liaise with the catering team to provide 'finger food' wherever possible for the resident, to help to maintain their dignity and nutritional well-being.

There has been much research around the use of coloured crockery. Home & Medical (2014) echo the findings from the two previous PEARL reports (FSHC 2013), suggesting that this has a huge benefit for some residents, and that staff therefore need to consider this as an option for residents on an individual basis where unexplained weight loss is taking place.

Coloured crockery also helps people who are at risk of losing weight, as food stands out better against a different background, allowing residents to see it better. This also facilitates a resident's independence. Initially blue crockery was used in our homes, but it was soon identified that certain food groups or types did not look attractive against a blue background, so as a company we now use the Dignity range of crockery, which includes a pale green and bright yellow.

Another big area of debate around facilitating independence is that of acceptable risk taking and allowing residents living with dementia to still be in control. Brooker (2007) says, 'There is often tremendous pressure to err on the side of caution with regards to situations that may include an element of risk' (p.74), and certainly from my experiences, I would wholeheartedly agree with this.

With the blame culture very much the 'in-thing', combined with at times over-zealous inspection regimes, staff often shy away from allowing residents to continue to do things they may have done the week before when they lived in their own home. So, for example, if a resident is still able to use a teapot or pour juice from a jug, then do we promote this and are these available on dining tables? The answer is probably not, in the vast majority of cases. However, when it comes to assessing risk we need to take into account the risk of not allowing a resident to maintain their skills and independence (risks on well-being, boredom, levels of frustration and helplessness). Therefore a measured individual approach needs to be taken, and where there are elements of risk from a safety perspective, then we need to look at ways of minimising these rather than taking a blanket approach and stopping them completely.

Other simple steps can often be taken to further promote independence at mealtimes, such as enabling residents to butter their own toast if they wish, and allowing residents to put sugar in their own drink, both things we take for granted yet we appear to prefer 'to do' for residents rather than 'do with'.

Snack boxes are a good way of ensuring that residents have access to foods outside mealtimes. Our homes have devised many innovative ways of ensuring food is on hand 24/7 and is placed strategically around the home so residents can either help themselves or staff are able to freely offer snacks to residents.

MAINTAINING DIGNITY

Maintaining a resident's dignity is yet again a basic human right, and often staff will act without thinking of the consequences of their actions and the impact on the resident's personhood. Kitwood (1997) states 'Personhood is a standing or status that is bestowed upon one human being, by others, in the context of relationship and social being. It implies recognition, respect and trust' (p.8). I actually find it shaming that 17 years on there is clearly still a need to inform some people in society about treating fellow human beings with courtesy and respect.

In relation to the mealtime experience, staff can promote a number of techniques and approaches to ensure that personhood is maintained.

Staff should assess each resident individually to establish if they would like some form of protection for their clothing, since clearly not all residents require this. Protection for clothing must be offered to any resident assessed as requiring this, but again, this must be an individual assessment, as some residents may only require or request a 'napkin', whilst other residents may require or ask for an apron or a tabard. Any form of protective clothing should never be referred to as a 'bib'; sadly there are still some 'child-like' aprons in circulation that are clearly infantilising.

Plastic crockery/cups should only be used for residents who have been assessed as requiring it (for example, if they have difficulty lifting heavier cups/plates etc.), and even when plastic is used, there are a number of items nowadays that have the appearance of traditional plates and cups. I can recall as a carer all residents drinking out of plastic cups because it was deemed as being 'safer'; however, as carers, we all had our own china or cups and mugs, and staff would often refer to the plastic cups as the 'residents' cups', as if there was a fear that dementia would be passed on.

Any resident who requires staff to cut their meal into small pieces to empower them to eat independently should consult the resident before this is carried out (or give an explanation as to why this needs to be done), and staff must address any unusual requests for food combinations sensitively, to avoid causing unnecessary distress (what the resident is requesting may be a preference they have always had and we therefore need to respect this individuality). As an example, a resident in one of our homes was losing weight and didn't appear to want any of his meals. When we got in touch with his son, it transpired that he would put tomato ketchup on every meal, regardless of what it was, and when we began to put ketchup on, he ate all of his meals and regained the weight he had lost.

Residents who may require assistance at mealtimes should have this carried out in a dignified manner and never be referred to as being fed by the staff team; any assistance should be afforded on a one-to-one basis.

Cultural diets also need to be respected within a care home environment, and homes need to be fully open and honest with residents prior to admission about whether they are able to meet these needs. To equip staff with this knowledge we have devised a dedicated section within our training package on some of the different cultural diets. However, staff must fully discuss these needs with the residents and/or their relative to see what aspects, if any, they choose to still follow.

Some residents may become distressed at mealtimes; however, this may be a result of the food they are presented with, frustrations that they cannot manage with the cutlery they have been provided with, or a feeling of disempowerment as they now have to rely on others to assist them. There may also be times that they do not get on with the person they are sat with; remember that as human beings we cannot get on with everyone all of time – this is just human nature…and not having a diagnosis of dementia.

EVALUATING THE MEALTIME EXPERIENCE

As mentioned earlier, there a number of ways in which, as a company, we currently evaluate the experience of our residents living with dementia during their mealtimes, wherever they choose to eat their meals.

Another tool often used to evaluate this experience is Dementia Care Mapping™ (DCM), as mentioned in Chapter 1, though for ethical reasons this is not undertaken within bedrooms.

Two observational extracts from DCM reports follow, undertaken during the lunchtime experience, showing how residents can experience both a negative and positive meal experience (residents' details have been anonymised).

Observation 1

During dinner, a resident was seated at a table that was facing the wall with another resident sat to their right.

The resident was given their dinner, though no choice was offered. The resident was clearly struggling to use the cutlery they had been provided with to cut up their meal. The resident ate some mashed potatoes, though after about five minutes they became frustrated at not being able to cut up their meal and in the end put the cutlery down. A carer removed the meal, assuming they had finished, and the resident proceeded to stare at the wall in front of them, disengaged from the environment.

Observation 2

At the beginning of the observation period the resident appeared to be quietly eating their lunch. The resident ate small portions only and remained in a neutral mood throughout the meal. They chatted intermittently with the other ladies sat at their table, but they didn't seem to want to engage in long conversations. Staff spent considerable periods with the resident, speaking to them gently, and ensuring that they had everything they wanted. The resident was offered a visual choice of meals, and staff gave them time to choose their preferred meal.

As a result of the PEARL programme (which also incorporates DCM, a quality dining audit, and relevant training) we have managed as a company to ensure that residents living with dementia can truly have a pleasant and enjoyable mealtime experience whilst improving their levels of nutritional intake and therefore benefiting physical health.

Analysis of data collated from 16 homes in the second PEARL study undertaken in 2013 (FSHC 2013) showed:

- Weight gain amongst an average of 42 per cent of residents in the participating homes, against the tendency for people with dementia to lose weight.

- Well-being increased amongst 46 per cent of residents. Well-being can be profiled against a set of measurement criteria including, for example, how the resident interacts, ability to communicate needs and choices, and having a sense of purpose.

As more homes undertake the programme, we can then clearly continue to improve or build on the mealtime experience for more residents living with dementia, whilst challenging the beliefs that mealtime is 'just another task'.

Chapter 7

Reducing Distressed Reactions

In this chapter, I explore whether most episodes of distress are avoidable, or at the very least, whether we can prevent episodes of distress from becoming unmanageable without the use of sedating medication. This chapter looks at how we can use non-pharmacological approaches that can help to reduce episodes of anxiety and distress. This is often referred to by many as 'challenging behaviour', but within the PEARL (Positively Enriching And enhancing Residents' Lives) programme we have purposefully lost this term to change the culture within the teams away from 'blame the resident' to almost self-blame. What did we miss?

> My stress tolerance is very low, and even a minor disruption can cause a catastrophic reaction, where I shout or scream, panic and pace. I need calm, no surprises, no sudden changes. (Bryden 2005, p.111)

And this is where our story starts. Daily life can be a struggle for people living with dementia in a care home. The environment is new, the people they are living with are new (and strange), the people looking after them are new (and strange). They cannot turn and see the faces of those closest to them. This is happening in a place that may already seem incredibly frightening as they struggle to try and make sense of the world within and around them.

Historically, we were trained to use an approach called 'reality orientation therapy', a technique initially used in the USA in the 1950s (Jacques and Jackson 2000) to help orientate a person to the current day and reality of what was happening around them. Whilst this has its place, particularly in the earlier stages of dementia, it can be incredibly frustrating for people in the middle to later stages of dementia to listen to or see things that may be in opposition to the world that they are currently experiencing.

A technique that seems to be much more appropriate is the use of validation therapy (Feil 1992), whereby the person working with the resident living with dementia is able to recognise and work alongside the resident's current reality, be that whether they think they should be collecting their children from school or carrying out their job as a postman. Most often, it is the underlying feelings associated with the subject of their experience. It may be that the resident is frightened, not sure or unable to remember what they should do next, and when staff talk through the underlying anxiety, often the distress is reduced. For example, a resident calling out for her mother may be seeking the comfort and reassurance of somebody she loves as she is feeling frightened or lost. Using reality orientation, we would have informed the resident that her mother is no longer with us. This might generally have two possible reactions. The resident might not believe you (as she believes her mother is still very much alive) and become cross with the staff member, or the resident may become upset as she is reminded of her loss once more.

Using validation therapy, the staff member would 'tap into' the experience and the underlying feelings surrounding the resident's request to see her mother. Staff would gently explore whether the resident was missing her mother, and perhaps ask what they would be doing if they were with their mother now. Often, the resident will take great joy in talking about her mother, and will perhaps recall childhood days or special occasions, giving staff an opportunity to expand on these and draw on the positive memories that the resident holds. Occasionally, the resident will come to her own realisation that her mother is no longer with them, but again, this affords the staff an opportunity to talk this through with the resident, acknowledging and validating her sense of loss.

Back in 2008, as part of our introduction to the programme, I wrote and read the following two extracts to the managers of the home, asking them to close their eyes and imagine that they were the person I was describing in the journey.

The first part of the fictional journey describes a fairly harrowing tale – a care home that might not understand how it could feel to be living with dementia:

The day has come that you have been dreading. You have known that it may happen for a long while now, but you have tried so hard to stay where you are, in the place that you adore…in the place that you lived with your family for so long.

You hear a knock on the door and you hesitate before you stand up. Perhaps you could change your mind, perhaps it's the milkman that you have known for 20 years coming to collect your money. No, it can't be – you paid him last week and cried silently as you told him that you wouldn't want any more milk – that you were going into a home. Your heart broke as he came in and you told him that you weren't coping since your partner had died. You remember his face, he was so sad, but he tried to joke with you, telling you that it would be a ball. You tried hard to believe him but your heart felt as if it was full of lead.

As there is another knock on the door, you cast your mind back to the other things you had to do last week, deciding which bits to put in your case. How on earth could you put your life in a case? You carefully choose pictures of the family, favourite clothes, favourite slippers, the picture of Goldie, your retriever, who was taken by a loving family (so the kennels said)…

You slowly move towards the door. A kindly lady looks at you, she shares your feelings, you can see that. Silently, you motion her through. You walk towards the back window and gaze into the garden that you have so lovingly tended for so many years. You look at the weeping willow and remember your grandchildren laughing and running in and out between the hanging leaves. You walk away from the window and look around your lounge, the lounge that holds so many lovely memories. Family gatherings, cosy nights in watching the television. Warm nights by the fire listening to the radio.

She picks your suitcase up, the kindly lady, and asks if you are ready. Your head is nodding but your feet won't move. She takes you by the arm and gently leads you to her car.

She tries to talk to you but you can't respond. You gaze silently out of the passenger window. Everything is rushing by, including, you feel, your life.

Too quickly, you arrive at 'the home'. She opens your door and again, you don't want to move. She helps you out of the car and you walk into what seems to be the reception. The kindly lady helps you to sit down and tells you she will be back in a minute. You are alone with your suitcase.

As you sit, waiting, you are aware of somebody screaming and you begin to get frightened. People in uniform start to rush past you, you smile, but they don't acknowledge you. You can hear noise, clattering. You want to go to the toilet but you don't know where they are, and you don't want to go off by yourself. You tell yourself that she will be back in a minute, the kindly lady, and so you wait, with a firm hand on your suitcase. You wait and you wait, you are desperate for the toilet. Somebody walks past – 'excuse me dear' but again, you get no response. You can't help yourself, you are frightened and you find that you have not been able to hold on to it any longer. You are mortified, ashamed and you don't know what to do.

The kindly lady appears again – she looks at you and exclaims 'oh dear'. She introduces you to 'Paula' who says will help you settle into your room. Paula takes your case and helps you out of the chair. You hear her mutter under her breath 'oh great' and then she calls loudly for somebody called Claire to come and clean the chair as you've been incontinent.

You are so ashamed, you apologise profusely...she is striding out in front of you and you are desperately trying to keep up. 'Here you are', says Paula, 'this is your room.' You look around at the empty space and wonder how on earth you can ever make this feel like home.

Paula takes over – she throws your suitcase on the bed and quickly unzips it. She takes all your clothes out and throws them on hangers. She shoves your jumpers in one drawer and your underwear in another. Your pictures, she places in a pile on the dresser. She puts your toiletries in the bathroom but takes away your razor.

As she is walking out of the door with your case, she tells you that dinner is in 10 minutes.

You sit on your chair and look around, you put your head in your hands and cry. Somebody passing the door hears you crying. 'Come now, it's nothing to worry about, come and have your dinner.' Embarrassed, you follow the girl and she takes you into what appears to be a canteen. Lots and lots of strange faces. She sits you down and puts dinner in front of you. Slowly, you eat the dinner, and as soon as you put your knife and fork on the plate, somebody who you can't see takes the plate away and bangs a pudding down in front of you. You lift your head and notice the commotion. Some people are being fed. Staff are rushing up and down scraping plates. Others are talking about the party they went to last night. The others like you though, look sad, very, very sad.

When dinner is over they take you to a 'comfy chair'. A chair amongst many in a large but very dull lounge. The television is on but nobody is watching it. Somebody comes to take you to the toilet. They at least notice you have wet trousers and take them off, but then they put these funny net pant things on and a great big pad. You try to protest and tell them that it was an accident, but they carry on anyway. They take you back to the lounge and you stay there until teatime, whereupon some sandwiches are brought to you with a cup of tea. Not long after tea, Paula comes back and tells you that she is taking you to bed. She leads you back to the room and starts to undress you – you try to tell her that you will do it yourself but your voice is lost. You lay in your single bed, looking up at the ceiling and around the walls, and again you begin to cry. Eventually, after what seems an eternity, you fall asleep.

The above passage should begin to help staff to recognise that whilst it is hoped that they do not associate with all of it, that they probably associate with some of it. This is not generally because staff are malicious, but because they are busy multitasking, thinking of the next thing that they have to do. However, staff don't always think about the effect that this might have on a resident living with dementia who might find it difficult to keep up with the pace of the staff. If a resident is being rushed, they will probably become more confused and upset. They may then become frustrated and angry (probably more at themselves), and then they may lash out or shout. Would this be 'challenging behaviour'? Absolutely not. This phrase has been reframed by some as 'behaviour that challenges others' but the term 'behaviour' remains, along with its negative connotations.

Christine Bryden describes this so well in her book. She believes that the term 'adaptive behaviour', where someone is adapting to a care environment, should be adopted (Bryden 2005). She goes on to describe many 'normal' situations within a care environment that occur, such as a resident spitting out their food because they don't like it, or going to the toilet in the wrong place because they have forgotten where the toilet is – things that might happen to a person living with dementia because they may not be able to articulate what they need, or remember where they need to be. Christine also has the vision to make it absolutely clear that if the care environment is focused on the person and their needs, then so-called 'challenging' behaviour would not occur (Bryden 2005).

After reading Christine's book, we originally decided to adopt the term 'distressed behaviour', but whilst giving the rationale to a group of care staff during a teaching session, one of them highlighted that we were still referring to behaviour and shouldn't we actually refer to this as a 'reaction' to a distressing situation? This made so much more sense as generally it was a reaction to things that we had (inadvertently) done or said or not done or said. Occasionally, distressed reactions may occur because the person living with dementia was responding to hallucinations of some form, but they were still distressed reactions, although it was an 'internal' influence as opposed to an external influence that we could affect.

We adopted the term immediately, and revised our policies and forms to reflect the term 'reaction' rather than behaviour, and for many of our staff, it was a light bulb moment. Almost immediately, we began to see a real culture change. However we had tried to explain this in the past, many staff still struggled with the concept that this wasn't just down to the 'dementia' and all it brought with it.

By using the term and framework of distressed reactions, it began to really help staff to reflect on their approach and to have a real empathy with the resident in the care home. Alongside this, we also taught resident experience training (Baker 2008), so that staff could have a greater understanding of how it might feel to live within a care home environment, both positive and negative. Staff are initially given a brief life story to complete prior to the training. They are briefed about the day and are asked to wear ear plugs, smeared sunglasses and to have their predominant arm immobilised. We also ask staff to wear a wet (with tap water) incontinence pad. During the morning, staff are assisted by the trainers to take their meals, move around, receive 'medication' and participate in daily care routines within the home whilst being exposed to aspects of mild malignant social psychology – for example, brushing their hair without prior warning or communication. During the afternoon, we work with the staff in a very person-centred way and work with their life story elements rather than against them. Staff are then interviewed about their experience and asked to translate their own experience into the care that the residents may experience on a daily basis.

As well as understanding the many facets of person-centred care and how this might influence the resident's experience, staff become very self-analytical: do I need to re-phrase this? Do I need to wait a while? Do I need to play some favourite music whilst we carry this out? They also become very proactive and use the information that they know from the person's life history, routine, choices, likes and dislikes to try and prevent them from becoming distressed in the first place (explained further in Chapter 11).

The second part of the narrative journey helps staff to focus on the introduction of person-centred approaches:

> When you wake up, the kindly lady is your room. She is apologising profusely…she says…
>
> 'I am so sorry, I brought you to the wrong care home. I will help you pack your bag.'

You get back into the car, with your lovely suitcase, so relieved to be getting out of there. She pulls up outside and helps you walk to the new reception. You are met by the manager of the home – she is very smart and has a very kind face. She recognises that you are upset and takes hold of your hand. She tells you a bit about the home and the sort of things that you could be involved in if you want to. She asks a lady called Mary if she could show you to your room. Mary, apparently, is going to be your key worker, a care companion, and will take special care of you. That feels such a relief. Mary takes your arm and walks with you to the room. Again, it looks a bit bare, but it feels different – warm.

Mary helps you to sit in the chair and then kneels down by your side and takes your hand.

She talks to you kindly and recognises how upsetting it is to move out of your house. She talks to you about your family and dog. She asks if she can open your case and help you to unpack. She asks you where you would like your things to go. She asks you where you would like your pictures, and stands them up on the dresser where you wanted them. She helps you to change your shoes for your favourite slippers, and asks if you would like a cup of tea.

She comes back with a cup of tea and some papers. She tells you that they are the menus for the day and asks what you would like to eat. She then sits with you and asks you a bit more about yourself as she would like to be able to share the information with other staff so that they can get to know you too.

A little later, Mary comes back and asks if you would like to go to the dining room. She points things out along the way so that you will remember how to get back to your room. This dining room is much nicer, it's like a restaurant. Lovely tablecloths and napkins – this is starting to feel much better. As you walk into the room, Mary asks where you would like to sit. You spot an older lady with a friendly face and ask if you can sit by her. Mary introduces you to Daisy and Daisy pats the seat next to her, inviting you to sit down. There is music playing softly in the background, nice relaxing music. Mary offers you a drink and goes to fetch your meal. It looks lovely. Lunchtime passes quickly as you chat to other people and laugh about your experience yesterday.

Mary comes to you after lunch and asks if you would like to go in the main lounge with other residents or go back to your room. You are actually quite enjoying yourself, so you ask to go to the lounge. She shows you in. A nice bright, airy lounge but really homely. The other residents are smiling. Some are knitting, some are reading the paper, some are listening to Glen Miller on the CD player. Mary asks if you would like a paper, but you decline, you are quite happy to listen to the music. You sit and look around, tapping your foot and tapping your fingers on the arm of the chair. Mary has shown you where the toilets are, but you can't remember. You see a member of staff – 'excuse me dear' – she smiles at you and asks how she can help. You tell her that you can't remember where the toilet is. She replies 'no problem, I will take you there myself.'

As she walks with you she tells you her name is Sharon and welcomes you to the home. When you get to the toilet door, Sharon asks if you would like any assistance. You politely decline and Sharon tells you that she will wait outside of the door so that she can show you the way back to the lounge.

Later on, in your room, a nurse called Julia knocks on your door. You call to her to come in and you see that she is carrying lots of paperwork. She sits by your side and asks if it would be okay to ask you a bit about your life and how you would like your stay to progress within the home. You tell her that you are worried about having a bath by yourself, and she reassures you that somebody can come with you. She takes a note of what you are still able to do and what you need help with. After she has written it all down, she asks if you would like to sign at the bottom of your support plan to confirm that this is how you would like to receive your care.

She then asks you about what you would like to do each day, what hobbies you have and how you would like to be involved in the home. She fills in another form and tells you that she will pass this on to the activities coordinator.

You spend the rest of the evening in your room, watching television, feeling really comfortable and at home.

At about 10pm, Amanda comes to see you and introduces herself as a member of the night staff. She asks if you would like any help getting into bed. You tell her that you are quite happy at the moment as you are watching a film, but ask her if she would pop back in about an hour as you might need a little help with your shirt buttons.

Amanda returns to your room at 11pm with a cup of Horlicks, and you are surprised that Julia, the nurse, has remembered. Amanda helps you with your shirt buttons and tells you to press the call button if you need anything else.

Your drink your Horlicks, and put on your nightclothes. You get into bed and close your eyes. You think about your house, but you are not sad, because you feel that this can be your new home without the loneliness that you felt before you came in.

The narrative above demonstrates how staff are seen to be working in a person-centred way, working alongside the resident, establishing their choices and respecting their independence and privacy.

If we are aware of the resident's preferred routine and lifestyle choices and work with them, it is less likely that the resident will become distressed. However, we all have days that we change our minds, and that should be okay too! If a resident is objecting to having a care task carried out at a particular time, we should respect their wishes and try again later. We all have the right to say no. The only time that we would work against this principle is if the person is in immediate danger, or at risk of ill health (or their privacy and/or dignity is compromised) if the care task was not carried out.

It can be really difficult for staff to work with residents in these situations when they are truly person-centred in their approach for a number of reasons. If we are truly person-centred, we should respect and accept the resident's wishes. However, if we know the person has been incontinent of urine, for example, and we ask the resident if they wish to accompany us to get changed and they say 'no', we are fairly limited as we don't want to go down the route of 'forcing' somebody to go with us. When we know our residents well, we also know that the person is likely to say 'no' if given a choice. We should therefore reframe our communication to reflect the need – for example, 'Okay then Fred, we need to take you to your room to get changed.' If the resident remains reluctant to come with us, we should acknowledge that, and assure them that that's okay, and try again a few minutes later, possibly with different members of staff.

When considering the reduction of distress, staff should also work with the family or friends to find out what the person is anxious about and generally what helps. They should also establish the things that bring the resident joy and that they are happy to talk about. Care plans should include this information along with any signs that staff have observed that lead them to think the resident is about to become distressed, for example, beginning to walk quickly, getting up and down from their chair, to enable staff to intercept and establish what is causing concern.

Obviously, distressed reactions are not always predictable, but staff also need to be mindful of things that may create a distressed reaction. By asking the following questions as we carry out care, we are ever mindful that if we don't pay attention to any of these things, the resident may become unduly distressed.

Communication?

Are we communicating clearly and at a pace so that the resident was able to receive our message? Do we need to re-phrase our message or request, and are we giving the resident time to respond? Are we speaking as an adult to an adult?

Involvement and inclusion?

Are we involving the resident as far as we are able? Are we including them in their care? Are we trying to keep them as independent as possible?

Environment?

Is the environment too noisy? Is the resident able to find their way around independently? Can the resident find a place to go if they want some peace and quiet?

Everything okay?

Is the resident in pain? Do they have a urine infection? Are they thirsty? (There is further information on this in Chapter 11).

Lifestyle and choices?

Does the resident want to do this now? Can it be left until later? What would they prefer to be doing now? Is there anything else or anybody else that they need to help them?

Memory impairment and self?

Is the resident feeling frightened because their memory is impaired? Do they recognise me? Have I explained who I am? Are they missing home? Are they missing family? Does the resident think they should be somewhere else?

The most important thing to remember about distressed reactions is not to blame. Don't blame the resident and don't blame ourselves. Sometimes, despite our best efforts, we will not get to the route of the distress. At these times, sometimes residents just want to be held, to be given 'permission' to cry, to tell them that they are safe with us.

We need you to reassure us and to be with us as a guide. (Bryden 2005, p.152)

Chapter 8

Reviewing the Use of Anti-psychotic Medication

Dr Pete Calveley

In this chapter, I look primarily at how we might begin the process of anti-psychotic medication reduction within the care home. There has been a huge government drive to reduce the use of anti-psychotic medication for many reasons that will be explained within this chapter. In order to reduce the use of anti-psychotic medication, the PEARL (Positively Enriching And enhancing Residents' Lives) programme has helped staff to look at alternatives and to look at episodes of distress that may arise for other reasons. Too often in the past, staff have turned to a GP for 'sedating' medication to help them out of a crisis, whereas in fact, sometimes the medication itself can cause further distress.

HISTORIC BACKGROUND AND CURRENT CONTEXT

There are almost 800,000 people over the age of 65 currently living with dementia in the UK. The incidence of dementia ranges from 1.5 per cent of those aged 65–69 to 23 per cent of those aged over 85 (Alzheimer's Society 2013a). Most people living with dementia will experience some form of behavioural and psychological symptoms (BPS) through the course of their condition, but often the opportunity to assess and manage these symptoms correctly will be missed. Since 2007 NICE guidance (National Institute for Health and Care Excellence), updated in 2010, has recommended that the first line of treatment for BPS should be psychosocial interventions (NICE and SCIE 2011), and that those should be improved with a tailored approach to the targeted use of anti-cholinesterase inhibitors, anti-depressants and analgesics. And yet, all too often, even today, anti-psychotics are often used as first-line treatment.

For several years it has been understood that anti-psychotic medications are both inappropriately and over-prescribed for people living with dementia. It is also clear that this inappropriate prescribing has both a very negative impact on the person's ability to maintain life skills and a positive interaction with the environment and those who care for them, and involves the use of powerful drugs with very significant side-effects including stroke, Parkinson's, falls and even death. Banerjee (2009) suggests, after reviewing the evidence for the use of anti-psychotic medications in dementia, that atypical anti-psychotics have only a limited positive effect in treating the behavioural and psychological symptoms of dementia but can cause significant harm. It was estimated that in 2009 around 180,000 people living with dementia (20 per cent) were treated with anti-psychotics per year, with only 36,000 deriving any benefit from the treatment (Banerjee 2009).

The Prime Minister's Dementia Challenge in 2012 built on the work of the National Dementia Strategy and had, as one of its core aims, a greater understanding of and research into both the cause of and effective interventions for people living with dementia with an expectation of an associated significant reduction in anti-psychotic prescribing. The results of recent research using the UK Clinical Practice Research Datalink (formerly known as the General Practice Research Database) showed a very encouraging reduction in the prescribing of anti-psychotics, which, by 2011, had fallen to prescribing in only 7 per cent of people living with dementia in the community (Martinez, Jones and Rietbrock 2013). Recent figures for the use of anti-psychotics in people living with dementia in care homes suggest that this may be currently at a level of 21 per cent of all residents (Shah *et al.* 2011).

The BPS experienced by an individual living with dementia include confusion, anxiety, tearfulness, agitation, walking around, shouting, physical and psychological distress and sleep disturbance. The dynamic of the interactions of the evolving dementia process itself, with other physical and psychological co-morbidities, is complex and not easily separated but is the cause of the symptomatology in dementia and, if better understood, can lead to much more focused and appropriate interventions that minimise the commencement and continued use of anti-psychotics.

Working with a person and focusing on the drivers of the BPS in dementia requires a skilled social, psychological and physical history and assessment, involving both the person and their family, and using evidence-based observational techniques such as Dementia Care Mapping™ (DCM) (University of Bradford 2005). Through this careful analysis and understanding of the person, a clear understanding of the drivers for distress can be gained, and a personalised plan for care, social and psychological support and, if necessary, prescribing, can be tailored.

EVIDENCE OF PHYSICAL HARM

Before considering the harmful side effects of anti-psychotics it is worth noting that there are many classes of prescribed medication whose side effects can exacerbate the symptoms of dementia. Anti-cholinergic drugs such as tricyclic anti-depressants, urinary anti-spasmodics such as Oxybutynin, bowel anti-spasmodics such as Mebeverine and Parkinson's treatments such as Procyclidine all work on the acetylcholine receptors in the brain that are already impaired in dementia. Side effects include poor concentration, drowsiness and memory impairment. Opiate analgesics can also cause sedation and confusion (Harwood 2013).

Whilst anti-psychotic drugs have a very real place for the treatment of co-existing psychotic disorders such as schizophrenia, and with people with psychotic symptoms and severe distress related to their underlying dementia, the prescribing of these powerful medicines should not be in any way routine, and should generally only be initiated under specialist advice.

The side effects of the use of anti-psychotics in dementia can be severe and are well documented by Banerjee (2009). For every 1000 patients with BPS of dementia treated with an anti-psychotic drug for 12 weeks, this would result in:

- an additional 91–200 patients with behaviour disturbance (or an additional 72 patients out of 1000 with psychosis), showing clinically significant improvement in these symptoms

- an additional ten deaths

- an additional 18 cerebral vascular accidents (strokes), around half of which may be severe

- no additional falls or fractures, and

- an additional 58–94 patients with gait disturbance.

Clearly this is very good evidence as to why the use of anti-psychotics should be restricted to only where other interventions are inappropriate or have failed and there is clear likelihood of benefit.

AN ALTERNATIVE RATIONALE

In order to reduce the use of anti-psychotic medication, the PEARL programme has helped staff to look at alternatives to sedative medication, and to look at episodes of distress that may arise for other reasons. In this section we summarise alternative reasons or exacerbating factors that may present with the BPS associated with a primary dementia diagnosis. When time and care is taken to understand the person and their unique situation, then alternative solutions and interventions may be attempted prior to resorting to the use of anti-psychotics.

Unfamiliarity and disorientation

When a person living with dementia is admitted to a care home, they will either have been removed from the familiar surroundings of their home and loved ones, or recently had a difficult experience in an acute hospital ward. In both circumstances it is quite normal to experience feelings of fear, anxiety, loneliness and uncertainty. It is often during an acute hospital admission that anti-psychotics are initiated to manage either delirium or an acute confusional state due to illness or disorientation. Unfortunately anti-psychotics are often not discontinued prior to transfer to a care home, and staff may not challenge this initially as they generally accept that they have been prescribed for a good reason. Rather than initiate anti-psychotics, a period of considered observation, calm reassurance and skilled interaction involving family, friends and professionals with a knowledge of the individual will often lead to a more comfortable and settled interaction of the person with the environment and staff.

Unmanaged or poorly managed pain

Symptoms frequently associated with people living with dementia are crying out, shouting, agitation and irritability, particularly when moving, dressing, bathing and during supportive or assistive physical care. There is well-documented evidence of the relative inadequacy of prescribing of simple analgesics (pain relief) in the elderly population living with dementia compared to a similar group without a diagnosis of dementia. It is clear that the painful conditions of osteoarthritis, osteoporosis, neuralgia etc. are equally common in both populations and yet, because a person living with dementia may not be able to explain, or complain directly regarding what may be widespread pain, we generally under-prescribe analgesia and prescribe anti-psychotic medications to manage their distress. It is important that we understand the physical, behavioural and psychological issues and needs of our residents, and ensure that a careful history, assessment and, if necessary, physical examination is performed whenever symptoms or behaviours may have pain as a underlying factor. A new report by Napp (2014) demonstrated that pain is under-recognised by nursing home staff who believe that less than half of residents living with dementia suffer from pain, when the nationally recognised figure for a care home population is 80 per cent. The report also suggested that guidelines for assessing and managing pain were under-used, and that less than a third of staff were trained in such assessment.

Frustration and anxiety

In the early to moderate stages of dementia people will have varying levels of insight into their condition, and may experience a range of emotions in response to their awareness of the progressive intellectual, emotional and functional impact that dementia is having on their own lives and the lives of those who care for them. These emotions can include denial, frustration, sadness, anger and despair. At the same time, the ability to exercise control and restraint of these emotions may also become less powerful, and behaviour may become less inhibited. This, in turn, can lead to further frustrations. As the condition progresses, the ability to communicate socially and express needs, fears and desires can become increasingly impaired, which together with any disinhibition may cause overt signs of pent-up frustration, verbalisation and distress if the fundamental need, desire or anxiety is not recognised by experienced carers or relatives. This is a key stage where, historically, staff and carers would request that sedating or anti-psychotic medication be prescribed. The importance of the elements of the PEARL programme that optimise the environment, provide appropriate stimulation, reassurance, calmness and therapeutic interaction and, in particular, focus on training and equipping the staff in person-centred care, the empathy of the resident experience and the personalised learning that flows from DCM cannot be over-stated if unnecessary and inappropriate prescribing is to be avoided.

Depression

There is no reason to believe that depression should be any less common in those living with dementia than those who are not. In fact, there are several arguments to suggest it should be more common. Many of the BPS of dementia such as tearfulness, sleep disorder, restlessness and agitation can also be presentations of depressive illness, and certainly one condition can co-exist with and exacerbate the other. For many years, however, the use of anti-depressants in people living with dementia was lower than should be expected, and anti-psychotics were potentially inappropriately prescribed where anti-depressants may have been more appropriate. The anti-depressants used currently are normally from SSRIs (Selective Serotonin Reuptake Inhibitors) so as to minimise the risk of side effects. Examples of SSRIs commonly prescribed are sertraline, citalopram and fluoxetine. The recognition of the under-treatment of depression has led to an increase in the prescribing of these anti-depressants, which, in the Martinez study, rose from being prescribed in 10.7 per cent to 26.3 per cent of a large cohort of 50,000 patients with dementia between 2007 and 2011. However, as research and clinical studies evolve, we must constantly re-assess our clinical practice. A recent Health Technology Assessment (Banerjee *et al.* 2013) found that two commonly prescribed anti-depressants failed to improve depression symptoms in patients with suspected Alzheimer's disease, calling into question NICE advice that those with a 'major depressive disorder' should be offered anti-depressants.

A PRAGMATIC, EVIDENCE-BASED APPROACH

PEARL is an evidence-based service built up from national and international research and best practice. We have incorporated within our learning the guidance in *Optimising Treatment and Care for People with Behavioural and Psychological Symptoms of Dementia* (Alzheimer's Society 2011), which supports the approach of observation and assessment to understand causation, with the use of skilled training and simple intervention and the need for patience, support and empathy before considering the use of specialist interventions and/or anti-psychotics.

When an individual living with dementia comes from home or hospital, where neither the environment nor the staff and carers have been through specialist configuration and training, and enters a PEARL home where the service and environment has been specially oriented and built around the personal, psychological, social and physical needs of that person, then it is not surprising that one of the key aims and expectations of the service is to minimise that individual's use of anti-psychotic medication to only that which is essential.

Within the PEARL service there is, however, no rush to reduce or stop medication of any sort – a person's prescribing history is bespoke to themselves. There will have been a specific reasoning, timing and trigger for the commencement of anti-psychotic medication, with the complex dynamics of the reasons behind this not always clear on admission. It is important to establish why the medication was prescribed through talking with the family, GP and, where appropriate, the hospital doctor or discharge liaison nurse.

It is important to allow the resident to settle in the home for a few weeks before attempting any reduction in medication, while using observation including DCM and well-being charts to understand the dynamics of positive and negative triggers to the person's emotional and behavioural balance. Family and staff are understandably nervous about altering medication that is perceived to have been prescribed for good reason, and may still be having beneficial effects, particularly if the anti-psychotic has been prescribed for a long time. It is important to involve the resident's family, care manager and GP in any discussion about altering or reducing medication, and to outline the intention to reduce and, it is hoped, stop the anti-psychotic in a controlled, supervised manner over an agreed period of time. Reassurance can be given that the medication can be re-introduced at any time if there are good clinical indications to do so. A large part of the process in reducing anti-psychotic medication is to increase the awareness of both staff and relatives of the common anti-psychotics in use, and the key side effects of the most common medications in use. Risperidone is currently the only licensed anti-psychotic for short-term use in people living with dementia (Alzheimer's Society 2013b).

Each resident living with dementia within a care home must have a regular review with their GP or consultant psychiatrist to discuss the necessity of any continued prescription of anti-psychotic medication. It is good practice to have a detailed care plan to demonstrate why the medication was prescribed, the side effects that it may have (so that staff can be on the look-out for these), and when it should be reviewed.

Within the PEARL programme, there has been an average 50 per cent reduction in anti-psychotic medication across the two phases that have been measured so far, with only a very small percentage of people having to be re-prescribed an anti-psychotic for a period of time.

Some of the anti-psychotic medications can increase confusion and will therefore increase dependency on others more rapidly and cause further distress for our residents. We must make every effort to provide non-pharmacological interventions for people living with dementia so that we don't create further complexities on an already very difficult journey.

Chapter 9

Developing the Environment

Providing a Supportive Environment

In this chapter, I describe what we have found to be helpful (and what has worked) within the dementia care environment. There are lots of ideas within this chapter that have really helped to 'calm' the environment and help people to find their way around the home. This chapter also looks at the types of activities that can be beneficial within the care home.

ENVIRONMENT

There has been much research surrounding environmental considerations within a dementia care unit, and many of the suggestions have been tried and tested within our programme. Some of them have been extremely beneficial and other recommendations have been 'adapted' as the original recommendation seemed to have little benefit. Other ideas within this chapter have come from experience of running a care home and working with people living with dementia and seeing 'what works'.

General signs

One of the most important considerations within a dementia care unit is the careful use of appropriate signage. We commissioned a company to provide bespoke signage that would contrast against the colour of our toilet and bathroom doors and reflect the colour of the toilet seat that we use. It is helpful to use both the word and picture of the room so that the resident is able to interpret one or the other or both. We have placed signage at eye level for the average height person, but I have also seen overhead flags used in other countries (USA and Denmark) within the corridors so that residents can see what is coming up, and I am informed that these work very well.

The signs do not have to be expensive, but they do have to be clear. Pictures need to represent the 'object' of the room as far as possible, and the text should be the same for all signs, bold and clear.

We advise that other signage is removed or placed out of eye line (at the top right-hand corner of the door) if it is necessary to keep it fixed on, for example, a fire zone number.

Bedrooms

There has been real debate about the use of different coloured doors for bedrooms within our own team. The argument for this is that the resident will come to know their own door and we may possibly be able to paint the door the colour of their previous front door. However, we have tended to move away from this concept for a number of reasons. First, if the corridors are narrower, it can drastically reduce the light. Second, it may represent the colour of their previous door, but if the resident associates with the home they had many years ago rather than their most recent one, this will not help and may in fact hinder. Third, 'their' (blue) door will be one amongst many in a larger unit; and last, to be able to use contrast for toilet and bathroom doors, we need to keep the remainder of the doors white or 'blended' (see Figure 9.1).

However, we can still make the bedroom door significant for the resident. The door should still have a bold number, and signage placed on it should focus on the resident's name (the name they prefer to be called) and a picture that the resident will associate with (in their younger days or perhaps a picture of a favourite pet). We tend to discourage letterboxes unless they are functional (i.e., you can post letters through them!) since although they can make the door appear like a front door, the resident may get frustrated trying to open the letter box.

Inside the room, we encourage the resident and relatives to bring in personal memorabilia that will facilitate conversation and provide comfort for the resident. Some of our relatives have put together terrific 'story boards' charting people's life stories and giving key pieces of information that staff can then use to chat to the resident whilst helping them with personal care or simply during a visit to the room (see Chapter 3 for more on this).

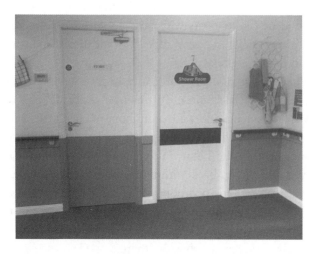

Figure 9.1: An example of a blended door

It is helpful if photographs can have dates and names on the back so that if the resident is unable to tell us who they are and/ or is becoming upset, we can use the information to prompt and guide.

We also encourage the use of portable memory boxes in preference to fixed memory boxes on the wall. Again the reason for this is twofold. Portable memory boxes can be taken with the resident into the garden or sensory room, for example, whereas fixed memory boxes, whilst helpful for orientation purposes, leave precious possessions out of reach, the resident being unable to touch or smell their treasured objects.

Residents may wish to have a CD player in their room and again, this can be particularly helpful to play music of the resident's choice during personal care or to facilitate conversation during a restful period.

DVD players can be equally useful. Favourite programmes can be watched and enjoyed in the resident's own room, particularly if the resident is not particularly sociable. There are also two great relaxation DVDs produced by A Sense of Calm© that may be particularly helpful if the resident is feeling distressed or for residents who need to spend time in bed, as visually, the DVDs are very appealing and the accompanying music is extremely relaxing.

Where possible, we try not to lock bedroom doors as locked doors can cause frustration. This can be really difficult as we know that residents will walk in and out of each other's rooms and sometimes put things in their own pocket that get deposited elsewhere within the home, but generally these things can be retrieved and placed back within the room at a later time. In a large unit of 20 plus bedrooms, imagine a resident trying all the doors and finding they are all locked, plus we use items and signage to orientate people to their room, so we don't want their room locked when they get there!

Toilets

We have tried various colours for toilet doors within our homes to help highlight its use, but found the most compelling colour for the residents was aqua green. During the pilot of the programme, we found that residents began to ask for 'the green door'.

To help to provide contrast, we use a blue-coloured toilet seat and railings (and this is featured on the sign), and we recommend that the wall behind the toilet was also painted in a contrasting colour so that the toilet is clearly distinguishable from the wall.

Bathrooms

Bathrooms can appear quite cold, clinical and mechanical when accommodating a specialist bath, and have traditionally been decorated with white tiles and cream flooring within our homes, to give them a nice 'clean' look. Residents can often become distressed during bathing, perhaps because the bathroom doesn't look like a traditional bathroom at home. Our staff introduced a homely feel to the bathrooms by applying suitable stencils or pictures on the walls, toiletries and bathroom ornaments on shelving, coloured towels and either voile or colourful blinds at the windows. Battery-operated CD players can be placed on shelving so that the resident's chosen music can be played during bathing, and battery-operated 'candles' can also be purchased to help to create a relaxed ambience and a more enjoyable bathing experience.

One of our residents loved watching one of the 'bath bombs' fizzing around and scattering petals in the water!

Corridors

Little can be done about the physical layout of the corridor in general, but much can be done to enhance the look and 'feel' of the corridor. Large stretches of corridor should be broken up with 'rest areas' where possible (see below), and corridors can be 'unitised' by colour and theme to help orientate the resident.

We have generally used dark pastel shades (such as sky blue) at the bottom half of the wall and a cream colour at the top of the wall. The colour aids orientation and the lighter top half of the wall enhances lighting, and ensures that any pictures or objects clearly stand out (see Figure 9.1, page 131).

We have 'themed' the corridors in many of our homes, again primarily to aid orientation, but secondly to provide stimulation for residents who wish to walk around the home. The objects can then be used either independently or in collaboration with a staff member. We have learned through the programme that it is much more beneficial to put things on the wall that can be removed (a process of gathering and replacing happens on the night shift!).

Pictures and objects surrounding a theme should be grouped into a particular area. For example, a garden theme may be used on a corridor leading out to the garden to act as another visual cue to help orientate the resident. The walls should not be too 'busy' but should provide key pictures or items that encourage activity and communication.

'Blended' doors and frosted glass

Whilst carrying out observations within the care homes, it became very apparent that locked doors can cause immense frustration, leading to unnecessary distress. Obviously, some of the doors within the unit have to be locked (such as the treatment room), but we needed a way of those doors becoming less visible. During the pilot, we began to 'blend' the locked doors in to the remainder of the wall, and found that the residents walked by them (see Figure 9.1, page 131).

We also noticed similar levels of distress when doors from units lead out into the reception – when residents saw people passing by, they would knock on the glass, calling out, but the people on the other side were unable to hear.

One gentleman who had been admitted on the day that I visited the home was extremely distressed. He was almost at a running pace and kept going to the glass; any attempts to try and communicate with him were futile as he was so focused on the reception area. Ordinarily, we may have assisted the gentleman into the reception area and had a walk around with him, but he was so distressed (and so new to the home) that I was concerned that he may leave the building. I asked the staff if they would find a curtain or duvet to put over the glass as a temporary measure, and the effect was almost instantaneous. The gentleman's anxiety reduced significantly, enabling me to take him to a chair, share a cup of tea and talk through his concerns.

Within most of our homes, we now either frost or use the stained glass film that you can buy to put onto glass that views out onto public areas. In some areas, however, fire officers have not allowed this when they have inspected, so it has had to be removed.

Rest areas

Sometimes it can be really difficult to encourage a resident to sit down and take some rest when they are walking around the unit. We developed small 'rest areas' and made them inviting rather than just a chair, to encourage the resident to take a break either alone or with a staff member.

Generally, we place a small table in an area with books or magazines, a jug of cordial and some tumblers, and in some homes, where this is sited by an electric point, we have some nice music playing.

The most creative rest area I have seen is in one of our homes in Scotland. This was a unit that was quite small but they wanted an area that the residents could go to other than the lounge/dining area, and so they took everything out of a recessed storage cupboard and adapted that! (Figure 9.2.)

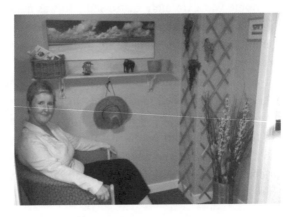

Figure 9.2: Home Manager Dorothy in the rest area created for residents

Lounge and dining areas

Dining areas have been covered earlier, in Chapter 6, but in general we try and keep the lounge area as homely as possibly without any theming. It is advisable to ensure that chairs contrast against the carpet colouring so that people do not 'miss' the chairs when they go to sit down. We have lots of sensory cushions – there are some great examples in the shops now that are furry or with raised embroidery. In some of the homes, we also have the lovely soft blankets that you can buy that either get wrapped around someone, held as a comforter or used to wrap dollies in!

Reminiscence rooms

In some of the homes that have additional lounge areas, the staff have created some wonderful reminiscence rooms (see Figure 9.3). I developed one in the care home I managed back in the early 1990s and the response was incredible. It not only provides residents with independent activity, but is also a great way to facilitate conversation and memories for both the staff and the relatives. The homes often find that they get overwhelmed with donations for the room, and they are in danger of becoming overcrowded, but items can be stored and rotated within the rooms to provide further stimulation.

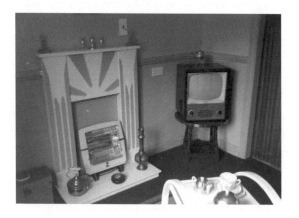

Figure 9.3: Example of a reminiscence room in one of the units

Sensory rooms

Again, I implemented one of these in the care home I managed back in the early 1990s and found that it really helped to reduce people's distress and provided a great forum for conversation. I carried out a small study at the time using Dementia Care Mapping™ (DCM), and found that we could use the sensory room in preference to 'as required' anti-psychotic medication when people began to become anxious or distressed. The equipment can be incredibly expensive if bought as a complete unit, but there are many outlets that sell sensory items now, and it can be great fun creating your own room with the residents!

The key piece of equipment that needs to be purchased from a recognised supplier is fibre optics as these have such great benefits for people and are very safe. The other key item that I would recommend would be the purchase of a bubble tube as again, the residents seem to find these very relaxing.

Garden area

Our care homes have various outdoor spaces as some are in cities with minimal land, and some are surrounded by fields but again, our staff have been very creative. In general, we need to make sure that the garden is as safe as possible to walk around independently and to have seating areas so that the residents are able to take a break.

There is a wealth of information around now to help you to plan a sensory garden, but the basic principles are that the residents can work safely in the garden (if they wish to), or they can relax and enjoy the garden or outside area.

In one of our care homes, the residents unfortunately looked out onto a concrete retaining wall from the dining room, and I can remember exclaiming what a pity it was, but the next time I visited, the concrete wall had been transformed! (see Figure 9.4.) I took the picture at this angle to demonstrate the tarmac path against it, but if you sat at the dining table, all you had was a beautiful view of the fields and hills with the sheep grazing.

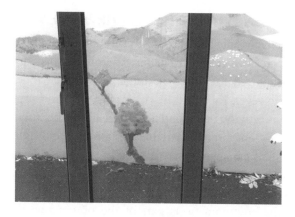

Figure 9.4: An external concrete wall transformed

In another one of the homes, the maintenance man came up with a really good idea to facilitate gardening activity for residents who were mobile and those who needed to use a wheelchair to get around. He put together raised planters that the chairs would fit underneath as he felt the concrete walled planters would still be difficult to access (see Figure 9.5). Note the drain cover that has been painted and made to look like a pond.

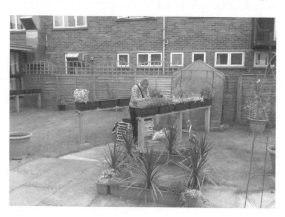

Figure 9.5: Accessible planters

ACTIVITIES WITHIN THE ENVIRONMENT

Being actively engaged is not for everybody, which is why we try and create nice environments where residents can simply relax and watch the world go by, if this is what they choose to do. However, for some residents, they like to purposefully engage in activity, but group activity may not be 'their thing'. It is really important therefore to create opportunities for independent engagement around the care home that residents can readily and safely access. For the purpose of this chapter, I focus on the activities or ideas that we have implemented within the environment as part of the programme that have demonstrated successful outcomes for the residents.

Doll therapy

The reaction to the implementation of empathy dolls has been outstanding (Baker 2009). Initially some staff (and relatives) were quite reluctant to use the dolls as they felt that it was treating older adults as children, a view supported by others (Mitchell and O'Donnell 2013), but once the staff observed the response to the dolls themselves, they were quick to change their minds.

I could really write a whole book about the positive responses we have observed, and we have had to be quite creative about additional needs that have arisen because the dolls have been introduced. For example, we have had residents who have not wanted to eat their meal because they have had to leave their doll, so the staff brought in a high chair for the doll to sit in – the dolls can get quite messy as the residents insist that they have a spoon or two as well! But the doll is taken away when the resident is soundly asleep, washed and tumble dried and back in their room before they know it is missing.

When I was carrying out an observation at one of the validations, I observed a lady who had four children, carrying out four empathy dolls, two in each arm. When she sat down, she placed them around her in her chair, and each one had a bite of the biscuit and a sip of the tea! She was chatting away, loving and cuddling them and kissing their noses – she was in such a high level of well-being, it was a joy to observe.

Another lovely observation I carried out was at one of our homes in Northern Ireland. A gentleman had begun to look a little bit anxious and distressed after dinner but the staff recognised this straight away and asked if they should fetch Charlie. I sat in wonder, waiting to find out who Charlie was, whether he was an animal or a friend or family member. Charlie turned out to be one of the empathy dolls, and the gentleman's face lit up when he saw him arrive and he immediately held him to his chest, wrapped his blanket around him and stroked his hair. Within minutes, he was totally relaxed and back in a good level of well-being.

I always feel privileged to work and observe in dementia care units, but some of the moments observing residents interacting with the dolls have really brought a huge lump to my throat. It is not for everybody, and a doll should be introduced gradually or left accessible for the resident to reach if they want to, but for those residents whose lives they have touched they have made an incredible difference.

Animals

Before considering animals within the dementia care unit, the staff need to ensure that a thorough risk assessment is carried out, both for the safety of the animal(s) and the residents and staff. There are some organisations that will bring animals into the care home, and these range from birds of prey, to reptiles to fully-grown donkeys!

Within our own homes we have had rabbits, birds, fluffy chickens, cats and dogs, but I think it has been the dogs that have had the most impact. In one home, the manager brought her puppy in from a few weeks old so that he could get used to the residents and the residents could interact with him as he grew up. The dog was extremely calm when he was with the residents (and was always observed during his puppy days), and when residents became poorly in bed, he would sleep at the foot of their bed or at their side, so that the resident could stroke him.

Within the same home, a lady had owned a fluffy white cat until it died of old age. She had its picture on her door (as an orientation cue) and she missed it terribly. The home purchased an animated fluffy white cat that would purr and move its head, and she carried it absolutely everywhere with her; it never left her side, providing huge comfort for her.

In a home in Scotland with an enclosed garden, the staff purchased a small bunny rabbit and allowed it to roam free during periods of the day as all of the units had full glass windows that looked out onto the garden. The bunny created havoc and uprooted most of the plants, but the residents would often be seen looking out of the window, laughing at its antics.

Again, animals are not for everybody, so the home needs to make sure that the residents living within it do not have any real fears about a proposed animal being brought into the home. A lot of our homes encourage relatives to bring in well-trained dogs so that they are only visiting for a short time.

Rummage boxes

Rummage boxes can be big or small and placed strategically around the home. Initially, we try to theme them so that they all contain items of a similar nature, for example, wedding memorabilia or childhood memorabilia, although they often get mixed up after a while! But they work as the name suggests. The resident is able to rummage around and select an item that grabs their attention, either to explore independently or to chat to someone else about.

Work stations

Several homes, where they have wide corridors and/or recesses, have set up small work stations that focus on a given area – for example, a handicraft area with accessible materials, an office area with an old typewriter and paper or a dressing area with a nice dressing table, its drawers full of necklaces and beads, scarves etc. Again, this is an independent activity that residents can choose to participate in.

Daily household living

Residents are part of the home and the home should revolve around the resident rather than the other way around. To help residents to feel at home, our staff encourage residents to participate in household life where it is safe and appropriate to do so (and the resident chooses to partake). For example, residents will help the housekeepers to dust, and will assist the maintenance man to carry out some sanding or painting. Residents love folding the warm towels straight from the tumble dryer. Setting tables, clearing tables, folding napkins – the home is a hive of activity. Often our residents have still led full and active lives before they come to us, and their many roles are left behind if we are not careful to help them to preserve their independence and identity.

Residents in bed

The clearest and most treasured memory that pops into my mind as I started to write this chapter was a lady who needed to be nursed in bed in one of the homes in the North East. The staff were not aware that we were coming (as we go unannounced to validate the home as a specialist unit). She was in need of end of life care and looked absolutely beautiful in her bed. She had her own 'cosy' blanket on, she looked immaculate, calm and comfortable and was gazing intently at the portable sensory equipment that the staff had put in her room.

After spending some time with her, I went into one of the lounges to read through some care records. The staff were unaware that I was in the lounge as this particular lounge was not often used by the residents. Every few minutes, as somebody walked by the room, they would call out to the lady and tell her where they were going or what they were doing or they would call into the room to have a quick chat and to see how she was.

It can potentially be a very lonely time for a resident if they need to spend all of their time in bed. However, there are many different forms of activity or engagement that we can use for residents in bed.

Sensory trays can be brought in to the resident for them to explore independently or as a joint activity with the staff (see Figure 9.6). The tray in the following picture was put together by a member of staff who initiated this for a lady who needed to spend a lot of time in bed. The lady took great joy from touching the various textures and talking about their use. She particularly liked the smiley faces! This was the first time I had come across this idea and I thought it was excellent and it was therefore cascaded across the organisation. The tray in question has a bean bag bottom so that it doesn't slip off the person's lap, and all of the items are very securely superglued on. Trays can be put together to reflect the resident's interests or life story, and it might be an activity that the relatives themselves would wish to do.

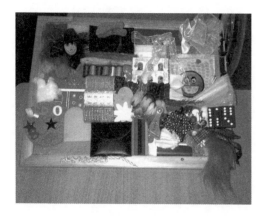

Figure 9.6: Sensory tray developed in a Scottish care home

Other staff within our homes will read poetry or books to our residents in bed, or they will provide gentle hand massages with the resident's own hand cream. Other activities could include talking through the resident's own life story book or through their photo albums, but sometimes all the resident wants is some company, somebody to sit and take hold of their hand whilst they rest quietly.

The key focus within any dementia care environment is to try and make it as relaxed and calm as possible. After all, there is enough confusion for the resident living with dementia without us contributing to it.

Chapter 10

Supporting Staff

Jason Corrigan

In this chapter, I focus on how we can support our staff to feel confident and capable in caring for someone living with dementia. This chapter provides an introduction to the types of learning that have been helpful to us within our programme, such as Dementia Care Mapping™ (DCM), person-centred care, person-centred planning, resident experience training, supervision and post-incident support.

Training for staff in any care home is essential to ensure that they not only have the skills, but also the confidence and competence to undertake their roles. Of course there are all the mandatory elements of training that staff require, such as health and safety, food hygiene, as well as training to provide the 'physical' aspects of care. However, in dementia care staff also require extra skills to be able to go that extra mile. By staff I am not just referring to carers and nurses – all grades and roles of staff require a certain element of understanding and awareness if we are truly looking to provide person-centred care. Despite this, I am always amazed when I read publications about dementia care and see that some providers still do not provide any training for their staff, or even see it as a priority.

Home from Home (Alzheimer's Society 2008) identified the need for training, and stated, 'While some of the personal skills required for good dementia care cannot be taught, good induction and on-going training are needed to develop a good staff team' (p.51), and four years later, the National Challenge (Alzheimer's Society 2012) still highlighted the need for dementia training for staff within care homes.

If a care home provided a service purely for people living with diabetes or, let's say, cancer, then you would expect the staff who worked there to have an awareness of that particular illness, how it can impact on someone, and how best to provide care for those individuals. Dementia care should be no different, and by this I don't that mean employing nurses will automatically address this issue. My work colleagues, some of whom are registered mental nurses (RMNs), others registered general nurses (RGNs), have informed me that dementia care is addressed briefly in the grand scheme of things during their nurse training, so the belief some hold (including some regulators) that as a nurse, you have been taught all there is to know to be able to deliver quality dementia care, is inaccurate. I am not pointing the finger of blame here at nurses, but am emphasising that to provide good dementia care requires compassion and specialist knowledge. In my opinion, dementia care is a specialism and should be respected as one by others. I also believe it is not a job just anyone can do. As well as the many various aspects of dementia care training that are needed to support staff (and I don't just mean the medical aspects), it also requires a caring, empathic and compassionate nature, and sadly some people just do not have this trait. Kitwood (1997) wrote, 'There seems to be something special about dementing conditions – almost as if they attract to themselves a particular kind of inhumanity' (p.14), and yes, we can educate staff around unintentional malignant social psychology and the impact on residents living with dementia that this can have, but as grown adults we usually know when we have either been intentionally rude or disrespectful, and so that is why it takes a special kind of person to provide true person-centred care. Sabat (1994) suggests that the way people are treated can result in behavioural and emotional difficulties, and this is another argument I would use to state that dementia care must be seen as a specialism.

I have always had a passion about training and ensuring that staff are properly equipped with the knowledge and skills to undertake their roles, and to also feel supported in what can at times be a stressful and emotional environment. Any employer has a duty of care to the staff they employ, and within the dementia care field this is no different. Person-centred approaches are required towards staff teams if in return we expect person-centred care to be delivered.

As mentioned within Chapter 1, the PEARL programme very much follows Dawn Brooker's VIPS framework of care, and this model places great emphasis on valuing staff. I now explain how we fulfil this, not only by supporting staff, but also by investing in them to become advocates for residents living with dementia.

E-LEARNING

This type of learning is becoming ever more popular within organisations as a way of providing staff with information. Within the programme there is a mandatory dementia awareness e-learning module that needs to be completed by all staff who work within the care home. The module itself covers five different sections in relation to dementia care, from the different types of dementia through to the importance of providing stimulation and meaningful activities, and each section has a set of knowledge questions at the end. This is a good way to introduce staff into the field of dementia care and to show how, within their roles, they all play a pivotal role, whether employed as handyperson, housekeeper, cook, activities coordinator, carer, nurse or manager.

E-learning in itself, however, is not the complete answer to educate staff to what I would deem an acceptable standard for working with residents living with dementia. It does not allow staff to ask questions, to challenge each other, build on teamwork or to learn from one another.

PERSON-CENTRED CARE TRAINING

As well as the e-learning module discussed above, all homes that start the programme are also required to send all members of staff (including home management) on a one-day 'Caring for Residents Living with Dementia – A Person-centred Approach' course. This mandatory course is for existing members of staff as well as new members of staff who join the home.

It is run by dedicated members of the Dementia Care Team within the company, and promotes staff to explore their own values and beliefs by providing a safe and open learning environment that encourages staff to challenge as well as learn. Staff are also provided with a resource pack that they can use to assist them further within their roles. This resource is aligned with a number of the company's specific dementia care policies and guidelines, and therefore encourages staff to further learn, ensuring a consistent approach is adopted.

The contents of the one-day course build on the information provided within the e-learning modules, and enable staff to explore and discuss what good person-centred care looks like in practice, the importance of relationship building and life story work, how residents may communicate their needs and how to identify and minimise distress, etc. Staff are also taught how to best use certain observation tools which, as a company, we find crucial in assisting in identifying levels of well-being or possible causes of ill-being in residents living with dementia.

I have seen many training packages over the years, and still today many companies offer person-centred training courses. However, when the contents of these are explored in detail, I still either see sections on 'challenging behaviours', or sections that refer to residents as 'sufferers' – they are not, therefore, truly person-centred courses!

As mentioned earlier in this book, as an example of valuing staff, many years ago during a training course a member of staff challenged the concept of behaviours, and said they felt that behaviour was a result of a reaction to some kind of distress. Ever since then, as a company, we now refer to behaviours as 'distressed reactions', which just goes to show that as practitioners and individuals we are always learning and should be open to learning from others.

PERSON-CENTRED CARE PLANNING

One area staff have always appeared to struggle with is putting their knowledge of residents down on paper. Nurses tend to like to write in the medical model, and carers like to write as it is; however, both sets of information are equally as important and both are required. It is about striking the right balance.

Over the past 30 years, the amount of recorded evidence required has certainly changed. I can remember as a carer in the late 1980s writing just one or two care plans for each resident. Oh how times have changed!

Another part of the programme is around documentation that is person-centred and inclusive (including the views and thoughts of the resident and their relative) – whether it's around personal care or meaningful activities. Listening to the staff teams within our care homes, we have devised a training course to enable staff to see what is actually meant by person-centred care planning, and how, from pre-assessment through to ongoing care planning and reviews, documentation can provide us with enriched meaningful information that ensures a holistic approach can be adopted at all times.

Labelling in relation to care documentation is another area that the training focuses on, and how by placing a label on residents we are in fear of not exploring possible reasons for their actions at times.

I have come across many 'labels' used over the years that sadly are still being used to date. In the table below I show you from my experience what staff have described residents as doing, and the label they have decided to attach to this.

Table 10.1: How we might label residents

What the resident was observed to do	Label used to describe their actions
The resident did not want to take their medication	Non-compliant
The resident pushed the carer away when they tried to assist them out of bed	Aggressive
The resident needs two staff members to assist them	A double
The resident needs a carer to assist them to eat their meals	Feeder
The resident walks around the care home	Wanderer

Clearly using terminology like this goes right against the promotion of person-centred care. However, this is a bigger area to address than that of just within the care home itself, as other health professionals and support staff are also just as guilty of using these labels on occasions, but by empowering staff to professionally 'challenge' others who use these choice of words, this is a start in the right direction.

RESIDENT EXPERIENCE TRAINING

Brooker (2007) informs us that 'Person-centred care is looking at the world from the perspective of the person living with dementia' (p.63), and therefore with this in mind, another part of the programme is a training course called 'Resident Experience Training' (Baker 2008).

This course is a very intense one-day course that requires up to two staff who are initially 'disabled' by being asked to put their predominant arm in a sling, to wear dark glasses so their vision is slightly impaired, to wear ear plugs and also put in place an incontinence pad. The purpose of this is so that they can experience what some of our residents experience due to their old age and frailty. Once these are in place, the staff are then exposed to elements of malignant social psychology – for example, they are assisted to eat at a fast pace, they are talked across as if they were not there, or ignored if they call out (these are often practices that staff sometimes do, either because they just don't think, or because of the culture of care within the home meaning that they are too busy focusing on the tasks).

Later on in the training session, the two staff are then exposed to person-centred care (prior to the course they are asked to provide a brief life story of themselves). This is then used to show inclusion, celebration and to provide a sense of acceptance amongst other person-centred techniques.

After the training and yet again as a way of providing support to staff, we provide a de-briefing session to explore the experiences with the staff to see how it felt for them. This element of the course is crucial, as sometimes staff reflect on their own practices, and it allows these to be talked through in a safe environment. (Obviously we are not talking about abuse here, but work practices that perhaps staff need to look at better ways of delivering and also ways of promoting inclusion.)

DEMENTIA CARE MAPPING TRAINING

DCM training, as mentioned earlier in Chapter 1, is an observation tool that was first introduced back in the early 1990s. Over the years there have been many of these tools introduced that have been reviewed (Brooker 1995); however, according to Kitwood, DCM provides us with 'A serious attempt to take the standpoint of the person with dementia, using a combination of empathy and observational and skill' (1997, p.4).

DCM has, over the years, become an internationally recognised tool to assist in the field of dementia care. Its purpose is to give us an insight of life in communal areas with the care home environment. It is an excellent way to observe and evidence how residents living with dementia spend their time, and how staff interactions can have an impact on their quality of life.

Within the programme we recognise the importance of such observational tools and the benefits they bring both to staff development and care delivery, and therefore we train a set number staff in each care home to become dementia care mappers. The course is accredited to the University of Bradford, and those staff members who attend also need to complete and pass an assessment to ensure they are competent in using the tool.

Once qualified, staff are then required as a minimum to undertake three hours worth of observations for three residents every three months, and to feed back their findings to the staff team as well as incorporating their findings into relevant care documentation to ensure that the whole team are aware of what may need to change or continue to be promoted.

As part of the DCM training, a section of the course focuses on how to feed back to others, especially when you may be bringing to their attention practices or routines that may need to be revisited. DCM should never be used as a tool for identifying individual staff and possible poor practices they may undertake, however – it is a tool for developing individual staff, promoting teamwork and looking at encouraging proactive ways of working, and whilst it may identify the need for certain training or change of work practices within a specific care home, it should not be used to make staff feel bad about themselves. With this in mind, when feeding back to the staff team it is important to seek their views and opinions so the mapper can explore with them why certain practices have taken place, or reinforce good practice that they may have observed.

DCM is also very valuable as a tool to assist staff if they are finding it hard to meet certain needs or to identify possible triggers for certain events. Each member of the Dementia Care Team within Four Seasons Health Care are qualified in DCM at various levels, and are therefore able to provide support and guidance to staff if ever they have any concerns or areas they are unsure about.

DEVELOPMENT PATHWAYS

For most staff the above training provides them with the skills and knowledge they require to undertake their specific roles within the care home in a person-centred manner and to feel supported to do so; however, some staff, including those who are new to the care environment, expressed a wish to further expand on their knowledge, and with this is mind, we have devised two development programmes, one for care staff and another for senior carers/nursing staff. These two programmes require staff to explore in more detail certain aspects of dementia care, for example, doll therapy, animal assisted therapy, promoting community links to name but a few, and certain elements of these two programmes have been aligned to the Skills for Care dementia pathways. This way, should staff choose to register for these awards, they will have already collated some evidence towards these.

Also within the project we look at regional/national opportunities staff are provided with, whether in-house or externally, and homes have become more proactive in resourcing what opportunities are available for their staff to build on their knowledge.

BESPOKE TRAINING

As well as the many training packages mentioned above, we have also devised a number of bespoke training sessions that are offered to staff within our homes. These courses have been developed when there may have been a need identified or a specific topic that staff required information and knowledge on to be able to ensure that they were meeting their residents' needs.

Examples of these include training on packages such as the Mental Capacity Act and best interests decision making, Deprivation of Liberty Safeguards, pain management in dementia care and abuse (physical, psychological, sociological and chemical).

As I mentioned earlier, I am very passionate about ensuring staff are equipped with the knowledge to undertake their roles; however, at times it can be hard for staff when they are provided with conflicting information on what constitutes good dementia care, information that clearly is just inaccurate, and when they are asked to undertake training that raises eyebrows.

These issues are often brought about by a lack of understanding in some areas by other professionals. For example, it is becoming quite common for some GPs or hospital staff to issue 'Do Not Attempt Resuscitation' (DNAR) documentation on the grounds of purely having a diagnosis of dementia, and this clearly goes against the principles of the Mental Capacity Act.

Another example would be that recently some regulators have been asking for staff in some of our care homes to be given instruction in 'restraint training'. Given the horrendous events of Winterbourne View (Flynn 2012), we would like to think that lessons had been learned. I appreciate there may be a need to act in a resident's best interest for certain individuals in extreme circumstances, and if this means stopping them from doing something because they would injure themselves or others (and they are unaware of this), then of course, we have a duty of care. However, situations like these need exploring in great detail and individualised measured approaches adopted. Using the word 'restraint' so freely is not the answer; adopting a person-centred approach is.

It is crucial for us to ensure that as a company we support our staff with any training requirements they need for them to be able to provide quality dementia care; therefore, whenever a new training need may be identified, it is essential to ensure that our staff are provided with the most up-to-date information. After all, our staff and residents deserve nothing less if we, too, are to be person-centred.

OTHER ELEMENTS OF THE PROGRAMME THAT PROMOTE SUPPORTING STAFF

Inclusion and involvement of the whole staff team is what underpins many of the criteria within the programme. I am a great believer that a home is only as good as it is managed, and a supportive manager will ensure that staff not only feel valued but also able to discuss concerns, share ideas and question practices when they are not sure.

Within the programme we seek active inclusion from the whole staff team involved, regardless of their role, as all the staff have an important part to play in ensuring quality care is delivered.

Regular support meetings and supervision are provided by a dedicated dementia care project manager, and whilst homes are undertaking the project, six-weekly visits are put in place to provide ongoing advice and guidance to staff, and also to answer any issues or queries they may have. Homes are also provided on each visit with six-weekly action plans that clearly set out what expectations are required, and this enables and promotes delegation amongst the different roles whilst under the leadership of the home management.

Staff are also supported to understand the VIPS framework of care (Brooker 2007), and each element is broken down so staff can see what this actually means in practice, and why it is important to all concerned. When changing the culture of care, it is vital that staff are fully aware of why changes need to take place and also involved and supported in promoting the changes. Failure to do so only means 'papering' over cracks, and bad practice will often begin to creep back in.

As I mentioned earlier, working in dementia care can be emotionally draining at times, and therefore teamwork and supervision is crucial to ensure staff do not feel 'burnt' out, so it is important that the staff team are also person-centred to one another, and do not unintentionally add pressures to their work loads. When I first started in care, staff would often undertake 'tasks' to please the next shift; for example, the afternoon shift would ensure all residents were in bed for the night shift and the night shift would return the favour and ensure most residents were up the next day, or the day shift would rush to get all the beds made by a set time or ensure all residents were up for breakfast.

Thankfully, as care homes begin to work towards the programme and staff feel supported and empowered, they soon realise that these are archaic ways of working and find it hard to believe that they actually undertook this approach in the first place.

It is important for staff to identify each other's strengths and to use these to further support one another; after all, we cannot be good at everything, and staff also have good and bad days, and that is where teamwork comes to the fore.

THE REWARD

The sheer look of delight on the faces of the staff when they have been successful at accreditation, added to a sense of pride and achievement, is priceless. We have heard laughter, seen tears of joy and lots of celebration parties, which makes the programme priceless. To see staff grow and develop over the programme is extremely rewarding, and even more so when the end result is a care home that not only provides excellent care, but also prides itself on delivering an excellent quality of care.

The specialist programme clearly promotes the importance of supporting staff and how in return, if you value your staff, then your staff grow and become more confident, and thus job satisfaction naturally follows.

However, don't just take my word for it; a number of statements follow from staff on their views on how the programme has made a difference to themselves and their care homes. (I have removed their names and replaced this with their job role.)

- A cook had noticed a considerable change in the care home since the programme began. They said it was a more colourful, comfortable, calmer and happier environment. They felt that they now think more about the care they provide to their residents living with dementia.

- A care assistant stated that the programme had changed their approach in dementia care as the training they had undertaken had really helped them, and now ensures that the care they deliver is the best it can be.

- A housekeeper informed us the because of the changes the programme promoted, staff have a different outlook and feel more informed and aware of the needs of residents living with dementia. The Housekeeper also felt that the environment was increasingly more homely and calmer, and that the management had empowered the staff team.

- The unit manager thought that over the period of time involved with the programme within the home, they had recognised that staff were less task-orientated and that staff were interacting with residents more, and also concentrating on residents being individuals and including residents more in making decisions and choices. They also believed that there had been huge changes in the communication between staff, and in particular, between day staff and night staff, and staff had also built better relationships with relatives.

When interviewing new staff for our Dementia Care Team, we always ask how they rate their knowledge of dementia care. We like to know that the prospective staff member has a sound knowledge of working with people living with dementia, but we always like to hear them admit that there is more to learn. Providing good dementia care is an ever-changing arena. We learn much from others and things that they have tried, but the people we learn most from...are our residents.

Chapter 11

Proactive Analysis and Follow-through

Sue Goldsmith

In this chapter, I provide an overview of what the care home should be monitoring, and how they should be monitoring their care – for example, reviewing the number of falls and distressed reactions, maintaining pain relief and weight, and what should be done if any adverse patterns are highlighted. This chapter will also include a focus on some of the specialist tools that might be used to provide proactive care that have not already been mentioned within the previous chapters.

Over the years, the role of the nurse and care worker has developed significantly. Gone are the days when it is enough to do as the doctor instructs, with little or no independent thought and input; now there is an expectation that nurses and care workers are knowledgeable, skilled individuals who are proactive in their thinking and, as a result, deliver a high quality of care for residents.

Throughout the programme, all staff are encouraged to rediscover that skilled and knowledgeable person who is often hidden away beneath years of doing things in a task-focused manner, to have the courage to question and to challenge, and to learn to work in a proactive rather than reactive way.

So how do we do this? The first step in achieving a proactive workforce is to enable and empower staff to work in this way. Brooker (2007) talks about the importance of valuing the individual, and believes that this also needs to be extended to the carer. How can we expect care workers to demonstrate that they value the people that they care for if they don't feel valued themselves? Valuing staff can take many forms. Although financial recompense is always welcomed, it is not always possible, so other ways of investing in staff should be sought.

'Knowledge is Power' was one of the most famous quotes of Sir Francis Bacon in 1597, and can be fully applied to the roles of care worker and nurse. An integral element of good quality dementia care is a well-trained workforce. The programme supports this ethos and endeavours to value staff by investing in their education and training as well as providing a platform for sharing ideas and listening to what the staff have to say. This is done in a manner that is non-judgemental and transparent, where staff feel able to voice any ideas, problems and concerns. As a result this has a positive impact on minimising the possibility of abuse, and serves to avoid a culture where poor quality care is accepted (Francis 2013).

The skill involved in analysing information that we gather is one that is developed through education and training. Encouraging staff to question and probe, to discuss and to delve ensures that they are continually looking to improve the quality of care that they are delivering to each resident.

SO WHAT ARE WE LOOKING FOR?

We can gain good insight into someone's quality of life if we analyse the information that we are presented with, even if the person is no longer able to tell us about their experience verbally. Quality of life can indicate to us whether the resident is receiving good quality care, or not, as the case may be. Due to the holistic nature of delivering good dementia care, it is not advisable to look at each element of care as an isolated event; instead, the whole picture should be observed, and recognition that one identified area of ill-being can have an impact on other elements of the person's life.

ANALYSING FALLS

Looking at possible causes of falls in residents can help to identify ways of minimising them. Encouraging residents to remain mobile can help to promote feelings of independence and self-confidence, therefore increasing levels of well-being. Remaining mobile can also reduce the risk of associated health problems including constipation, deep vein thrombosis (DVT) and chest infections. It is important for staff to be aware of several risk factors when considering why a resident might experience recurrent falls. According to Rubenstein (2006), these risk factors include:

- environmental factors such as loose rugs or mats, wet surfaces, lack of handholds
- low weight
- urinary incontinence
- polypharmacy
- diabetes mellitus
- cognitive impairment

- disturbed vision

- gait disorders

- ill-fitting footwear

- disturbed balance or coordination

- alcohol abuse.

Dementia is a particular risk factor as those experiencing visuospatial impairment may be at higher risk of falling. (Kröpelin *et al.* 2013, 549–563)

Already within this list of possible risk factors, we can observe other avenues that may need exploring. For example, if a resident is losing weight or is taking a number of medications to manage pre-existing conditions, these areas will also need to be addressed. Looking at issues in isolation will very rarely bring about a satisfying resolution; after all, we are complex creatures!

So what is the scope for prevention of falls? Addressing each of the risk factors identified above, we at least have a starting point for considering possible causes. Sometimes I see falls risk assessments that have been completed but not analysed. The information has not been used to formulate an effective care plan to minimise risk, and has therefore merely become a paper exercise. Staff then become almost accepting of falls, and become reactive bystanders rather than the proactive practitioners we wish to see looking after residents in our care homes. As well as considering the identified risk factors, staff should also look at any patterns that have emerged with any previous falls. Consider if the falls occur at a certain time of day or in a particular area of the care home. Are the same people present? Is the resident always wearing the same footwear when the falls occur? Just by thinking about these details staff could go a long way to identifying factors that may contribute to a fall. It may be that the person is more tired at a certain time of day, or that the falls occur following administration of a certain medication. It may also be that the falls occur in a part of the care home where the lighting is poor. With regard to others being present, could it be that the resident has become the target of another resident's frustration, fear or anger, possibly walking into their room looking for company or looking for their own room? Misinterpretation of intentions can lead to a manner of reactions, and may lead to a resident being pushed over by a fellow resident. If falls are occurring at night time, again, any patterns need to be looked for. Is the resident falling because they can't find the en-suite? If so, would it be an idea to leave the bathroom light on and the door ajar? If any of these causes are suspected, it is important that they are written into the care plan along with clear guidelines as to how these should be minimised. It may be that closer support is needed at certain times of day or when the resident is walking through certain parts of the building. It may mean that a resident needs assistance and further visual orientation to find their room, to avoid inadvertently walking into another person's room. Each reason will be very unique to each person, and staff should therefore be encouraged to 'think out of the box' in looking for these reasons.

The cause of falls can be multifactorial, therefore a multi-disciplinary approach is often required. Involving a GP to review medication, a dietician to improve diet, physiotherapist or occupational therapist to look at appropriate exercises to promote balance and gait are just some examples of other agencies that can help to be proactive in discovering the cause of falls. Multi-disciplinary falls teams are also present in most trusts now and are happy to visit and advise (NICE 2013).

Another significant risk factor in falls in older people is the prescription of hypnotic and psychotropic medication. In line with the National Dementia Strategy (DH 2009), the PEARL programme has asked staff to question why residents may be prescribed such medication, and to take an analytical approach in considering whether other medication, such as pain relief, may be more appropriate. This is discussed in depth earlier, in Chapter 8.

ANALYSIS OF BEHAVIOUR

With this in mind, analysis of behaviour is also a key factor in understanding the person and ensuring that we are doing everything possible to provide good quality care. Very early on within the PEARL (Positively Enriching And enhancing Residents' Lives) journey we ask staff to consider distress as a form of communication. Although this has been considered in depth earlier in Chapter 7, I think it is worth revisiting this again in terms of a proactive analysis.

Many of our residents are no longer able to express their displeasure, frustration, anger and irritations in the standard verbal manner, but this does not mean that their feelings are any less real! As a result we may see this manifest itself in other ways, and it may lead to residents being labelled as having 'challenging behaviour'. This instantly has a negative connotation and can lead staff to think that it is a result of a particular diagnosis, and therefore that they can do nothing about it. In reality, as we have seen time after time throughout the PEARL programme, referring to this as 'distress reactions' rather than 'challenging behaviour' promotes an analytical approach, and helps staff to adopt the mind set of there being a reason for the reaction, and therefore something that we can do about it.

For a number of years now the most common approach to establishing the cause of distress has been the 'ABC' method. This focuses on three elements that, when put together, can help to identify triggers and patterns to distress. Looking at the antecedent (A), viewing the resulting behaviour (B) and observing the consequences of this (C) helps staff gain a rudimentary insight into why our residents have sometimes acted in a particular manner. As part of the programme, we took this model and looked at the work of the Newcastle Challenging Behaviour Service (Newcastle Support Model; see James and Stephenson 2007) in order to see whether we could develop this basic ABC model to be a little more person-centred (i.e., to lose the label of challenging behaviour primarily), and to encourage our staff to be more inquisitive in their approach. As a result we developed a 'Distress Reaction' monitoring form that asks staff to probe into what has happened, but also asks them to focus more on the feelings and emotions that the resident was expressing at the time. In addition, asking staff to be mindful of the time of day and who was present at the time also helps staff to drill down to real possible root causes of distress, with a view to preventing the same circumstances from occurring again. This format also asks staff to reflect on the situation, and to think about what went well and what could have been done differently that may have resulted in less distress being experienced by the resident; this approach can gently remind staff that their approach and response to residents can have an impact on the outcome of a situation, and has been incredibly useful as a development tool as well as a tool to lessen the incidents of distress.

When asking staff to complete 'Distress Reaction' monitoring forms we also prompt them to complete additional observations and therefore consider other reasons why the resident may be distressed. We ask them to complete the Abbey Pain Scale to see if the cause of their distress is pain, the Cornell Depression Scale to consider whether they are showing signs of depression, and the Well-being Profiling Tool to see whether there are signs of ill-being. We also ask staff to consider other signs of physical ill health – are there any signs or symptoms of an underlying infection? As mentioned earlier, it is not enough to look at each piece of information gathered in isolation. Putting the clues together can often guide staff to making a correct assumption, and therefore putting the correct measures into place to resolve the situation. For example, a high Abbey score, together with a high Cornell score and a low Well-being score, may indicate that the person is showing signs of depression and ill-being because they are in pain. Addressing the pain may then result in the signs of depression being alleviated and well-being restored.

When considering distress experienced by residents, we also have to consider the dynamics that may exist between residents. In reality, the majority of our residents will be strangers to each other and before coming to live at the care home will not have encountered each other. Is it realistic therefore to expect everyone to like each other and to get on all of the time? I think this would be most unusual and would cause me to be quite concerned if residents didn't feel comfortable enough in their own home to express themselves or to do what they wanted. However, at times, dislike of someone or something that they are doing can manifest itself in distress and put residents at risk; it is therefore important that staff are attuned to the likes and dislikes of each resident, including people. Again, information following a 'resident-on-resident' incident should be analysed. Think about what was happening at the time, who was present, what was said and what the reaction was. As an example, did Doris hit Betty for no reason or because Betty was continually shouting 'Help' and Doris was not able to stand up and walk away? Staff need to analyse information like good detectives in order to be able to find satisfactory solutions for all parties concerned. In the above situation, staff should try to find out what is causing Betty to shout for help – is she frightened or lonely? Is she asking for a drink or to use the toilet? They also need to consider if Doris is feeling alright – does she dislike loud noises? Is it unusual for Doris to react in this way? In which case, if this reaction is out of character, staff should consider whether Doris is feeling unwell or is in pain. The outcome of reflective sessions should be documented within informative risk management care plans that highlight the distress reaction, possible reasons for it and measures that can be taken to minimise the risk. These plans need to be 'living' documents that are consulted and amended if further incidents occur, or if incidents reduce. Staff also need to accept that they might not find the solution immediately, but should continue to share ideas until an acceptable solution is found.

We also need to think about behaviours that are not intrusive but that may also be an indication of ill-being, and look at reasons behind why residents feel like this. During training sessions I will often ask staff, 'What would you do if a resident was running around the care home, singing and dancing and swinging from the chandeliers for long periods of time?' Staff always laugh and say that they would not think that this normal, would be concerned that the person was unwell and would probably consult the doctor. I then ask, 'What would you do if you saw a resident sitting quietly, not engaging, head in their hands, not smiling for long periods of time?' This is often met with silence as staff realise that what I am alluding to is that this is not normal either. But would we call the doctor? Possibly not – if the resident is not 'causing any problems', we may then write in their progress notes that they have had a 'settled day'. Settled for whom? For staff or the resident? However, it is incredibly important that we recognise that this type of behaviour can be an indication of a number of problems. Again, it is important to use our observation tools to ensure that we are monitoring closely for the possibility of pain or low mood. We also need to consider isolation, boredom, loneliness, fear and very importantly, the possibility of abuse and the impact that this can have on the quality of life of each resident. Knowing our residents will help us to determine what is out of character for that person and deter us from putting everything down to the progression of the illness.

During the programme we have also asked staff to analyse other behaviours that they may observe, behaviours that they may struggle to make sense of and are therefore in danger of accepting as a direct result of dementia. These behaviours have included taking clothes off in communal areas and smearing faeces, and I have delivered many heated and interesting training sessions that have resulted in staff coming up with some sensible and credible reasons for why a particular behaviour might be occurring. Listening to staff discussing the situation with each other in detail, agreeing for the most part but also disagreeing until a possible new approach is found, is both encouraging and refreshing. Returning a few weeks later and hearing staff proudly telling me how the behaviour has stopped and how the well-being of the resident has improved is excellent news. Of course, this isn't always a simple process and staff may not always get it right the first time; as I tell them, it is often a case of deduction, and not getting it right in the first instance should not be viewed as failure. It is only when we stop trying to find a solution to a problem that we can say that we have failed the person in our care.

Case study

Mrs A had lived in the care home for several months and had maintained her independence. She had a kind and loving family who visited twice weekly. Mrs A needed very little assistance from staff to attend to her personal hygiene and elimination needs on a day-to-day basis; she took great pride in her appearance and was pristine about hygiene.

However, after a few months, staff noticed that Mrs A was becoming less independent regarding her elimination needs and was occasionally incontinent of faeces. This caused Mrs A much embarrassment and she would try to attend to her hygiene needs following an incident of incontinence without the staff knowing. Staff assumed the reason for this was the progression of her dementia and would do their best to assist her with her hygiene needs following the event.

Mrs A was introduced to me during a visit to the home. We sat chatting for a while, and Mrs A talked with much pride about her children. She asked me where they were as they had gone without telling her when they would be home and she was worrying about them. I was unsure where they were, therefore told Mrs A I would go and find out for her as she was clearly worried. I found a member of staff who had got to know Mrs A very well, and the staff member told me about Mrs A's obvious attachment to her family and also about her health and life in general. She raised the subject of the occasional faecal incontinence, and made a passing comment that this only seemed to happen when her family had visited and staff had started to think that Mrs A was protesting about her family leaving without her. However, the staff member also told me that this would be out of character for Mrs A as she was not an objectionable person, but they couldn't think of any other reason for this. I gathered another two members of staff together and the four of us sat down and discussed possible reasons for this in depth. We looked at the circumstances that were occurring when the incontinence happened, who was present and what was actually being said. The outcome of the conversation was that it occurred directly after Mrs A's family left. The family were so intent on not upsetting Mrs A when they left, that they did not actually inform her that they were going home and when they would be back. This corresponded with the anxiety that I had come across when having a conversation with Mrs A earlier on in the day. We discussed how this could be making Mrs A feel, how it might cause her anxiety levels to increase to the point of her becoming incontinent. I asked the staff to think of a situation in the past where they had felt nervous or anxious, with 'butterflies in their stomach'. Each staff member could relate to this feeling and said that there was a great possibility that Mrs A was feeling like this when she didn't know where her family was and she was waiting for them to return.

It was agreed at this time that the nurse would discuss this with the daughters during their next visit, and would ask them to tell their mother when they were leaving and when they would be back. In addition, they would also ask the daughters to inform the care staff when they were leaving in order that they could then go to Mrs A and spend some time with her rather than her being alone. Staff were enthusiastic and keen to incorporate this immediately into her care plan in order that all staff were aware of what they were going to try.

When I returned to the home a few weeks later, the staff were keen to tell me just how successful this approach had been. They told me that Mrs A was much more relaxed after a visit from her daughters now because they told her they were leaving and when they would be back. The staff had observed that she was much less anxious and they could easily engage with her about her visit; in addition, they would use this opportunity to reinforce that her daughters had gone home and would be back to see her on another day, soon. Occasionally Mrs A would ask the staff to show her where the toilet was but, more often than not, she would be content to sit and chat and would not need the toilet. As a result of this, Mrs A no longer experienced episodes of incontinence, and it was therefore a successful outcome for all concerned. Mrs A's dignity and independence was maintained, and staff felt incredibly proud of how they had worked this out and put steps in place to find a solution.

ANALYSING PAIN

To analyse behaviour without considering the very real possibility of pain may very well result in unnecessary suffering on the part of the resident. The result may be in the form of distress, weight loss, disengagement, depression, decreased activity and disturbed sleep patterns (Horgas, McLennon and Floetke 2003). Any one of these issues may then lead to other associated problems that staff may then need to address, during which the resident's level of well-being is also negatively impacted on.

Throughout the programme we have reiterated the need to monitor pain levels of residents with all staff. A baseline medication audit will often highlight low levels of prescribed analgesia or pain relief that is prescribed on an 'as required' basis that is very rarely administered. When asked, staff often say that they will ask residents if they are in pain during medication rounds, and if they state that they are not, then staff will give no further thought to the need for pain relief. My flippant response to this is to ask staff whether they also ask residents if they are psychotic prior to administering an anti-psychotic drug; although a little harsh, this is usually enough to get staff to realise that paying brief attention to the real possibility of pain in this manner is not enough – proper and consistent observation by all staff is a much more satisfying approach.

It is now becoming increasingly recognised that pain experienced by an older person is often untreated, and the severity of pain can also be underestimated. Studies have concluded that this is more common for people who are living with dementia and, as a result, the prescription of effective pain relief is likely to be less than for those older people who do not have a cognitive impairment (Morrison and Siu 2000).

Advanced disease state or chronic conditions are common in older people, and it is important for staff working in the care home environment to recognise that these existing conditions also need to be continually monitored and treated in order that the person living with dementia is afforded the best opportunity for optimum well-being. Dementia does not supersede existing conditions, and therefore pain relief can have a huge impact on the course of the disease. On too many occasions, I have observed ineffective pain relief that would never be accepted for a person who is able to verbalise articulately that this is not working. An example of this was for a lady who was in the very advanced stages of bowel cancer who was prescribed paracetamol four times daily. In any other group of citizen, this would be deemed as scandalous and may even result in a public outcry, but sadly, for older people living with dementia, this is all too often accepted.

Throughout the programme, staff are taught and encouraged to be proactive in their attitude towards pain management. The first step is to establish whether the resident is in pain, and to aid with this we ask staff to use the Abbey Pain Scale (Abbey *et al.* 1998). This includes key behaviours representative of the scope of behavioural pain indicators in people with dementia. However, the tool also includes items such as physiological changes and causes of pain; these are not behavioural pain indicators, but add further factors to consider when assessing whether a person with dementia might be in pain. Staff in the care homes are asked to be very flexible in their approach when using this tool, and are asked to complete it on admission and then monthly thereafter (unless pain was suspected, in which case it should be carried out sooner). If it indicated that a person was in pain, we would ask that they take steps to alleviate the pain; this may include helping the person to reposition, applying heat to the affected area or administering analgesia. Staff are then asked to monitor the effects of this by repeating the pain assessment a little time later. Ensuring that staff continue to repeat this until the pain has diminished is integral to effective pain management as, too often, the attitude is that pain relief has been given, therefore what more can be done?

During the programme we observed that with this change in staff understanding came a change in the style of prescription of medication as we saw the use of anti-psychotic medication decrease and the uptake of analgesia increase. Staff reported individual cases where they observed complete changes in behaviour, increases in appetite and improvement in mood. As a result, for a large number of residents, anti-psychotic and hypnotic medication was gradually discontinued; prescriptions for food supplements also decreased and residents became more active and more involved in their own care.

ANALYSING WEIGHT LOSS

As mentioned in earlier chapters, historic thinking has been that people living with dementia will lose weight as a natural progression within the disease process. Within those chapters it is also explained how this shouldn't be another of those areas that is merely accepted by staff, as there is much that we can do to minimise the possibility of weight loss. The first step with this is to establish cause.

Staff should think about pre-existing conditions that may be the cause of weight loss; these may include cancer, diabetes or thyroid disease, and it is important that staff are aware of the signs and symptoms of these illnesses in order that they can monitor any associated complications. In the early stages of dementia, residents will often be able to tell staff if they have dental pain or difficulties in swallowing, and cause may be easier to establish. Staff should also be aware that depression is common in the early stages of dementia, and that this can cause loss of appetite and subsequent weight loss. It is important that mood is monitored, and this is discussed in more detail below.

As dementia progresses, residents may experience weight loss for other reasons. These may include an inability to focus or concentrate on food, or an inability to make verbal choices or express that they don't like the meal that is being served. Residents may also lose the ability to recognise food or everyday eating utensils, and staff need to be vigilant in recognising this so that they can offer appropriate support. As described in Chapter 6, the importance of enhancing the dining experience isn't solely for enjoyment, but also to try to minimise these issues and therefore to minimise the risk of weight loss.

Maintaining weight, hydration and nutrition is essential in a bid to maximise well-being of our residents living with dementia. Failing to do this can lead to so many associated problems that can further affect well-being and also lead to further dependence on care staff within the care home environment. Weight loss can lead to muscular weakness and this, in turn, can increase the risk of falls or increase physical dependency on staff, leading to a direct impact on well-being and also on the use of staff time. Ironically, this can mean staff become more task-focused at a time where residents may need more psychological support.

Lack of proper nutrition and hydration can also enhance the symptoms of confusion and disorientation. I remember a time in my life when I was incredibly busy and stressed with a full-time job and two small children. As a result, I started to neglect my diet, and this began to have an impact on my cognitive functioning. I would forget that I had done things such as locking doors or turning the washing machine on, and I even forgot who I had arranged to pick my (then seven-year-old) daughter up from school, which caused me much panic and anxiety. The final straw was when I got into the car to go to go to work and couldn't remember the way, despite having worked at the same place for two years. Frightened and convinced that I had a chronic cognitive impairment, I visited the GP who was very empathic and took my concerns seriously. Following a blood test, it was discovered that my poor diet had depleted my body of essential B vitamins, which was leading to my poor cognitive functioning. This made me realise just how important it is to ensure that my residents have a vitamin rich diet if they are to be given the best opportunity to live well with dementia.

ANALYSING MOOD

We can't describe ourselves as proactive practitioners if we don't give daily consideration to the mood and feelings of our residents. All of us strive to give our residents the best quality of life, but how do we monitor this?

Throughout the programme we have encouraged staff to use their observation skills and to question and analyse what they see. We have introduced the use of depression and well-being tools in order that they are able to monitor mood levels, and also to give some guidance as to what to do if anomalies are identified. Together with the knowledge of the resident, staff are then in a better position to try to identify cause of low mood or ill-being, and to look at ways to minimise this. The importance of recognising depression in a person with dementia is self-evident in terms of improved diagnosis and recognition of a potentially treatable condition. Most depression scales are completed with information provided by the person – something that is not always possible in cases of dementia (Alexopoulos *et al.* 1988).

During the programme, we introduce staff to the use of the Cornell Scale for Depression (Alexopoulos *et al.* 1988). This is a tool that is used to assess whether a person living with dementia is experiencing clinical signs of depression. It is based on observation of staff and knowledge of the resident, rather than solely from information gained verbally from the resident, as this is sometimes difficult to fully ascertain with a resident living with dementia. The analysis of the depressive symptoms does not change with this tool; merely the way the assessment is carried out is different. When carrying out this observation tool, we ask staff to complete this, ideally in small groups, as we have found that different staff members will observe different things. This helps staff to put a fuller picture together and therefore to gain a more accurate insight into how the person is feeling. Similarly we ask staff to complete the Well-being Profiling Tool (Bradford Dementia Group, University of Bradford). Profiling well-being is a formal way to put ourselves in the shoes of a person with dementia, and to work out how they are feeling. As dementia progresses, people may become less able to tell us how they are feeling. Using well-being profiling enables us to gather information over time to establish if the person we are caring for is maintaining well-being. If the profile shows that the person's well-being is deteriorating, it will give staff an opportunity to discuss the possible causative factors and to implement new strategies to maintain or improve well-being.

Both observation tools are completed regularly for each resident with the aim of highlighting changes promptly, giving staff a more structured approach that they can discuss with confidence with GPs if necessary. The use of the tools is also effective when monitoring the effects of anti-depressant medication, and again allows staff to have a formal evidence base for further discussion with the GP if needed.

Another invaluable tool in assessing well-being of individual residents is the use of Dementia Care Mapping™ (DCM). Throughout the programme, we try to ensure that there is at least one trained dementia care mapper in each home working towards accreditation. We ask that mapping takes place, as a minimum, on a three-monthly basis, and that any findings are discussed with the team and used to influence care planning. This tool has proved to have a wealth of benefits as it highlights areas of good practice and engagement as well as identifying areas that could be improved on. As a newly trained mapper some years ago, I attended a local authority strategy meeting following a resident-on-resident safeguarding incident. One member of the panel described DCM as a 'time and motion tool', which caused me much frustration and anger. The rest of the meeting was taken up with me explaining the benefits of DCM and giving examples of how my observations had had a direct positive impact on resolving the situation between the two residents involved. DCM is a tool that can allow the trained mapper to analyse what a resident is doing and how they are feeling, minute by minute. By focusing so closely on the person staff can identify subtle changes in facial expressions, movements and behaviour that in an everyday working environment may be missed by staff going about their daily work. These may be expressions of pain, discomfort or low mood (as a few examples), and combined with analysing mood and engagement levels of residents at the same time, this has proved time after time to be very accurate in pinpointing what causes well-being and ill-being. Of course, like any other information, this is only of use if staff take the time to implement findings and analyse on a regular basis whether the measures are having a positive impact on well-being. The tool can also identify the individual resident's reactions to interactions with others, and the mapper can help to identify preferences that residents have; this can be incredibly useful to know when it comes to trying to minimise any embarrassment or distress that may be experienced during personal care support.

Analysis of all that we see and all that we do is critical if we are going to continually offer the best possible care for our residents. All of the tools that we encourage staff to use are a starting point for analysis; however, they are only used with success when staff apply their skills of observation and break down the information that they have gathered. Accepting that each person living with dementia is a unique individual who will experience different levels of health and different emotions throughout the course of their life helps staff to ensure that they adapt their approach and their thinking accordingly. The adoption of an open-minded yet inquisitive approach helps staff to break away from the historic excuse of 'they do that because they have dementia' and instead look beyond the words or the behaviour to truly try to understand what the person is experiencing.

Chapter 12

Celebrating Success

In this chapter, I provide some insights from our residents, relatives and staff as to how the programme has made such a positive difference, and offer some thoughts as to how a care home might take the next steps to becoming a Centre of Excellence for People Living with Dementia.

There is no better feeling in the world than being present at a successful validation! Being able to see how the unit has developed over a period of 12 months, and the pride that the staff have taken in their work. Carrying out the observations, seeing such rich and skilled interactions with residents and feeding that back to the staff, who are often equally emotional and absolutely thrilled that their hard work and increased knowledge has had such a successful outcome.

Often, when I am carrying out Dementia Care Mapping™ (DCM) as part of a validation, I feel extremely privileged that I am able to witness such incredible care and the impact that it has on our residents who are being encouraged to live within such a positive home-like environment. Our residents are allowed to 'be' whoever they are, ensuring that distress is kept to an absolute minimum, and opportunities for positive engagement are increased to the maximum.

Of course, not all homes go through on first validation, and that can be really difficult for the staff to accept initially, but they often have an increased determination to make sure that they absolutely get it right. One home we worked with that was unsuccessful at validation (mainly around documentation) worked so incredibly hard over the next eight weeks on their action plan that they achieved Silver level at their subsequent validation. Most homes will achieve Bronze level at first validation, but in subsequent validations with further knowledge and experience, they will go on to achieve Silver or Gold levels. We were asked to introduce a Platinum level a couple of years ago (95% of score excellent) as we had 10 Gold level homes that wanted to achieve even more.

There are four distinct areas that have positive outcomes through the programme, and I wish to highlight some of the key successes as follows.

GREAT OUTCOMES FOR RESIDENTS

At the beginning of the programme, we send a data sheet for staff to complete around a number of key clinical outcomes. This same audit is then repeated (resident by resident) one month following the successful validation of the home.

Our biggest success by far has been the reduction in anti-psychotic medication, which averaged 52 per cent in Phase 1 of the programme and 48 per cent in Phase 2 (FSHC 2013). There were many reasons for this, and we need to do further analysis to establish if there are any specific trends to account for the reduction, but our 'sense' feel is that it mainly due to staff understanding that residents will sometimes call out because they need something (but are unable to articulate it), or they are uncomfortable, embarrassed, confused and frightened but certainly not 'challenging'. Medication is no longer a first-line response but a carefully considered option following a full review of the resident's needs and a variety of different approaches to understand any possible reason for the distress.

An increase in activity and a drive to maintain or promote independence seems to be the underlying success for an average 30 per cent reduction in depression scores amongst residents following the successful implementation of the programme. Again, further studies need to take place to look at the possible correlation of the approaches that we have implemented, but with staff more able to recognise possible distress or pain, this has undoubtedly led to an increase in well-being on average of 46 per cent.

With the introduction of mealtimes as an activity and an increased focus on how to support residents who may be at risk of losing weight, including the use of coloured crockery and naturally fortified meals, we recorded that 42 per cent of our residents on average experienced an increase in weight. Further work needs to be carried out to establish if there is a direct correlation with the reduction in depression scores along with a reduction in pain scores, or if these residents in particular were those who had their anti-psychotic medication reduced or discontinued.

On average, 42 per cent of the residents involved in the study were able to have their hypnotic medication (medication to help people sleep) discontinued. Was this because they were more active, more content, less anxious, less distressed? Along with this, we recorded that falls had reduced by 32 per cent on average amongst the residents whose data we captured. Again, there may be a direct correlation as residents were not so sleepy from medication that they had been taking.

Incredibly, 40 per cent of residents on average also had their medication to reduce their anxiety discontinued or reduced, which I firmly believe is because the staff were able to work with the resident in such a person-centred way that their anxiety was lessened.

The full details of the clinical outcomes can be found within the PEARL (Positively Enriching And enhancing Residents' Lives) report (FSHC 2013), but for now, let's hear some real resident success stories.

As each home goes through the programme we ask them to complete an evaluation and to provide comments about particular areas. I also emailed the homes last year when I knew I was going to write this book to ask staff if they would provide small case studies to demonstrate how the programme had worked particularly well for them in their home.

Case study 1: Susan (North East, England), by Pam and Helene, personal activity leaders

For the purpose of this case study we shall refer to our resident as 'Susan'.

PEARL was already in place when Susan, our 75-year-old resident, first arrived. Susan is mobile but is very cautious because of very poor vision, and still enjoys an active life where she feels part of our vibrant community.

Susan has regular family visits and enjoys socialisation, whether this is through music, outings or pampering sessions, and she also loves community involvement, whether externally or in the home.

Susan enjoys sensory stimulation, both within the PEARL-enriched environment and our gardens. Susan's senses are enhanced by the feel of the sun and the different scents of the flowers when outdoors. She is also positively stimulated whilst out shopping and on minibus outings to explore her surrounding environment. The musical instruments on the walls of the PEARL corridors encourage Susan to engage in sing-alongs to guitar, singing and dancing. She also loves the tactile feeling of the fabric flowers on the walls, which are garden themed. The Hollywood, beach and memory lane corridors also provide stimulation for Susan.

All of our staff benefit from resident experience training with special consideration to living with dementia. This has given our staff greater understanding and empathy, which benefits both staff and residents.

Case study 2: Care home (North, England), by Annette Banks, dementia care project manager

The home is now an Accredited Specialist Dementia Care Home, which has a 29-bedded residential dementia care unit. Prior to commencement of the programme, the dining room on the unit was very dull and uninviting, with no specific orientation to mealtimes.

Staff did not see the point in setting tables, and saw the tables being set as a risk, as residents may pick up the knives and forks and hurt themselves or others. Because of this, tables were not laid for meals, and residents were not offered the use of condiments.

Residents would come through to the dining room for their meal, but many did not stay and would get up and go back into the lounge or their bedroom, and meals would be served to them in those areas. Mealtimes were never seen as a celebration or a communal time for all.

Since the programme commenced, the dining experience became a focus to improve, and this started with the education of staff about the importance of making the dining room warm, homely and inviting. The dining room has been enhanced with bright-coloured pictures of food items such as cupcakes; each table now has a main tablecloth and an overlay cloth, and each place is set with a place mat, cutlery, glass and serviette.

Condiments are available on every table and a choice of sauces depending on the meal. There is a picture menu available and this is updated at the end of each meal; the chef or catering staff attends the unit and serves the meals. The options are plated up and then staff take both options to the resident to choose what they would like. For those residents who choose to eat in the lounge or bedroom, meals are offered on a tray that is laid with a doily, a serviette and cutlery, and residents are offered the choice of a clothes protector if they wish. Residents now come to the dining room and stay there for their meal, and everyone sees the importance of a good dining experience. Mealtimes are now a real celebration, and this has not just changed the life of one resident, but every resident within the unit.

Case study 3: Mrs A (Northern Ireland), by Yummy Hechanova, sister

This report outlines the behaviour of Mrs A before doll therapy was implemented in the unit, and the impact of introducing it to Mrs A.

Mrs A is 93 years old and diagnosed with dementia. She loves singing praising songs, but easily gets tired and bored. She can display distress reactions to staff, other residents and relatives, but every time staff tried to reassure her, she ends up crying. Staff tried all the activities they could think would benefit Mrs A, but unsuccessfully. However, when doll therapy was introduced to the unit, it made a huge impact on Mrs A who started holding and cuddling the dolls, and looks so content sitting in the lounge. Sometimes she talks to the doll and fixes its clothes and from then, it is evident that the incidence of Mrs A displaying distressed reactions has dropped.

Relatives' support is also very good wherein Mrs A's daughter brings clothes for the doll so she can change it when needed. At first, everyone might think that giving an older person a doll is so childish, but after implementing, it came out that it is a symbolic representation that helps the person living with dementia meet the very important emotional needs. Mrs A finds comfort in the doll and for her, it is the reality, and REALITY is all that matters for the person with dementia.

No one can just take it away from her or replace it, as to do so may lead to a distressed reaction.

If we can use doll therapy to assist residents during times of distress, then we can rely less on the medicines being given to 'calm them down'. By then, we will be enhancing the person to express what they feel, we will be respecting the person's dignity and we are maintaining the attachment of the person to something as it is vital for a person with dementia living in long-term care.

GREAT OUTCOMES FOR RELATIVES AND FRIENDS

Within the majority of our homes, friends and relatives of our residents have always been willing to take an active part in the resident's care. For some, this helps to provide continuation of a role they took prior to the resident coming into the home, which we actively encourage as, however good we are, we will never know the person as well as they might.

However, I feel that I must share a story here to demonstrate that as a relative, we don't always know best! When visiting my own grandmother in hospital, I was appalled to see that she had been given a plastic beaker with a lid on it. My grandmother was quite 'well to do', she had been fortunate to have tea with the Queen, and constantly reprimanded me and my brother as children for not curling our little finger when we drank our tea out of her bone china cups, so you can imagine my horror. My immediate thought was that they were not at all person-centred, that they had not taken into account any element of her life story, and that she was being treated like everybody else. Trying to keep the frostiness out of my request, I asked the staff if they could kindly transfer her beaker of tea into a cup and saucer, as my Nan would not appreciate a plastic beaker. They looked at me a bit strangely, but met my request and gave me the cup of tea, which I took to my Nan's bedside. We sat for a while chatting, and then I asked her if she wanted some of her tea as it was going cold, to which she replied 'Oh I thought that was for you dear...I have to drink it out of that plastic beaker so I don't spill it down myself.'

That taught me such a huge lesson!

Our relatives have really helped us to develop some fantastic life stories that we are able to use as an activity with the residents. Some relatives have created amazing life story boards, depicting family trees and achievements. One of our homes worked with the relatives to produce some incredible life story DVDs which were so useful as they also had residents' favourite pieces of music playing in the background. As part of the validation, we interview relatives or friends where we are able, and it is so heart-warming and humbling to hear of relatives feeling safe and secure in the knowledge that their relative is placed within the home. One particular lady will forever stay etched within my mind as she described one of our homes as a lifeline a couple of years ago. This lady's husband actually came as a day resident as there were no day care facilities. The lady had come to the end of her tether as her husband was being quite sexually active; she felt that it was because he was in his reality of many years ago. As an older lady herself, she could not keep up with him, but loved him dearly, and didn't want to him to go into a home full time at that time. She told us that he had been so much better at home since he had been attending as a day resident, and that she had been able to stop his anti-psychotic medication. I saw her again a couple of months ago. Her husband is now living in the care home but she is happy in the knowledge that he is being well cared for.

And the words of another relative will also stay in my mind. This was a home that, when I carried out the baseline data, 92 per cent of the residents were taking anti-psychotic medications (and are now down to 17 per cent):

My husband had been in bed for 16 months. In a matter of weeks at the home he was up and about. On the next visit we sat in the lounge eating breakfast together and he is much more aware and alert. The only medication he is on now is blood pressure tablets. It is remarkable.

GREAT OUTCOMES FOR STAFF

And we can't forget the staff. We have witnessed incredible creativity and a sense of ownership throughout the project. Home managers are absolutely key to ensuring that the project is a success, but staff within the homes have taken ownership for micro projects, and have formed committees to theme walls, gather all the life story information, make the dining experience a much better one and deliver the resident experience training to each other. Initially staff were concerned that to deliver truly person-centred care they would need many more staff, but quite quickly came to the realisation that actually, if they were all working in a person-centred way, the job became easier as there was less distress and anxiety to overcome. Staff talk about having much more time to spend with the residents to complete activities and to simply chat. Studies on the staff turnover figure have shown that there is a 30 per cent reduction in turnover in the homes where the programme has been implemented.

As an example, here is an email we received (copied to the Senior Management Team and the chief executive) early last year following a home that had been re-accredited from Gold to Platinum:

Hi Everyone

It is with great pride that I am sending this email, the proud manager of the most dedicated, caring, compassionate and professional team of staff that I have ever worked with.

The team here at (the home) are ecstatic today now that they are over the initial shock and are already gathering in the home for a team celebration, with residents and relatives, and a smile beaming Regional Manager.

The dedication of the staff here to maintaining PEARL has always been evident and I am so pleased for Noreen and her staff, who maintain this standard each and every day, and in the words of the accreditation team true person-centred care.

It is also with great pride that I can say, I am very proud to work for a company that supports its staff and homes through PEARL, in developing Dementia Services to ensure that our residents are treated with the dignity and respect that they deserve.

Sincerely

Heather Lyttle

The following is an evaluation completed by a home manager whose team achieved a Bronze level award:

PEARL EVALUATION: MANAGER'S PERSPECTIVE

Please answer as fully and as honestly as you can to help us to both evaluate the project but to also to shape the future of the project.

Looking back to the beginning of the project, how do you think your dementia care unit faired in relation to how it is now?	I thought that we were providing good care and had good working practices, until we started with PEARL.
	The project has made both myself and staff look at our practices and each other's and we are now able to critique ourselves in how we approach residents. We have a greater understanding of residents through life stories. These have helped massively in providing more person-centred care and activities. We now have a 'what's best for the residents' approach rather than 'what's the easiest way for staff'.

Do you think the project has made a big impact on the dementia care unit? Please explain your answer	Yes. In all aspects.
	The environment – the themed corridors are enjoyed by staff, residents and visitors. They are a great source of reminiscing.
	The lounges are comfortable and pleasant. But I feel that biggest achievement with the home is the dining experience. We constantly tried to make the residents' experience good, but we just weren't achieving this. We tried numerous ideas, e.g. two sittings, but together we came up with setting up two dining areas downstairs and this works really well. Mealtimes are now calm and relaxing.
Have you found that the person-centred care training has been helpful? If so, please give examples	Yes – again it made us look at how we speak to residents and how we label people without intending to offend. I listened to staff after doing the training and realised how many labels we had – the walkers, the feeders, the turns.
	It has changed our thinking, but we have to be careful not to avoid one label and giving another in its place.
	It also helped in the way we write our care plans. On reflection, the care plans we had contained a lot of negative statements about our residents – e.g. aggressive, resistive or uncooperative. We worked well as a team to word our care plans more positively. Every time we came up with a good care plan (or so we thought) we would share it.
	I myself became more involved with writing care plans.

Have you found that the DCM training/use has been helpful? If so, please give examples	Yes – we have a resident who the family think is unhappy and does not like it here (at the home). We mapped her and during her six-monthly review spoke to the family that said they thought she was unhappy.
	This lady's mapping indicated that 90% of the time she was in well-being; we established that although she does not engage with conversations with other residents, she likes to just listen and also that when music is playing in the background she was tapping her foot along to the music.
	Even if you aren't mapping it has made us more sensitive to how residents may be feeling.
Do you think that having a project manager to support you has helped you with the project? If so, please give examples	Absolutely – you need someone to guide you and point you in the right direction. Jason gave ideas e.g. how to enhance the themed walls, how to improve the care plans, he was there for advice by email and phone – I never had to wait any length of time if I had any queries. He was there for moral support too, when I felt that we weren't going to achieve PEARL in the timescales we set.
Please detail any other support that you have received to help you attain your PEARL award	As mentioned above – also from Sandra Shaw RM. She supported me throughout, she was conscious too that I felt towards the end that I wasn't going to achieve PEARL in the timescales set. Rather than failing, she would have supported me postponing – but I'm glad we didn't!!!!!!!!
How do you personally feel about achieving your PEARL award?	Very proud, both of myself and staff. I have a great team, and I felt that they were on board in achieving PEARL. I have a good team and they deserve to be recognised for their hard work and commitment.
How do you think your staff feel about achieving the PEARL award?	I think they feel proud too. Their commitment has paid off. We did well!

My computer is full of similar evaluations. As you will see, pride simply oozes from the home manager and the team, as well as most staff, reflecting that although they felt they did a good job beforehand (and they did provide great fundamental care), they have a real sense of accomplishment that they are now providing specialised dementia care for the residents living within the home.

GREAT OUTCOMES FOR THE REST OF THE ORGANISATION

As the programme has progressed, we have seen that homes that have not started on the programme as yet have started to implement parts of the programme independently. The results of the programme have been presented at our conferences, and our staff recognise that the programme is really valuable and not simply a 'tick box' exercise.

I have spoken at many conferences in England, Chicago, South Africa and Taipei, and I was always asked if we could give out a copy of the criteria. As I mentioned at the start of the book, the criteria need to be developed against the organisation's own ethos and policies as it is so important that it has ownership from board to ward and the other way round. What I did promise, however, it that I would write a book, a book that will, it is hoped, help staff within the care homes to implement some of the practices and ideas that we have outlined.

There have been many people on this journey with us – a true collaborative process, and that is the key. None of this would have happened if there was any break in the chain. Support and commitment to achieve excellence in dementia care at every level has resulted in a programme that has changed so many people's lives in such a positive way. We have been extremely fortunate and been able to secure dedicated staff resources to help to progress the programme, but any small change can make such a significant impact.

A care home will never be the same as the person's own home, but we can do so much to try and make it feel like their own home and that they belong.

> The precious string of pearls, of memories, that is our life, is breaking, the pearls are being lost. But by finding new pearls, those created in the struggle with dementia, we can put together a new necklace of life, of hope in our future. (Bryden 2005, p.170)

PEARL – Positively Enriching And enhancing Residents' Lives

References

Abbey, J.A., DeBellis, A., Piller, N., Esterman, A., Parker, D., Giles, L. and Lowcay, B. (1998) *The Abbey Pain Scale*. Mooroolbark, Australia: Dementia Care Australia Pty Ltd.

Alexopoulos, G.S., Abrams, R.C., Young, R.C. and Shamolan, C.A. (1988) 'Cornell Scale for depression in dementia.' *Biological Psychiatry 23*, 3, 271–284.

Alzheimer's Society (2008) *Home from Home: A Report Highlighting the Opportunities for Improving Standards of Dementia Care in Care Homes*. London, UK: Alzheimer's Society.

Alzheimer's Society (2011) *Optimising Treatment and Care for People with Behavioural and Psychological Symptoms of Dementia: A Best Practice Guide for Health and Social Care Professionals*. London, UK: Alzheimer's Society.

Alzheimer's Society (2012) *Dementia 2013: A National Challenge*. London, UK: Alzheimer's Society.

Alzheimer's Society (2013a) 'Demography.' Available at http://alzheimers.org.uk/site/scripts/documents_info.php?documentID=412, accessed on 3 February 2014.

Alzheimer's Society (2013b) 'Antipsychotic Drugs.' Available at www.alzheimers.org.uk/site/scripts/documents_info.php?documentID=548, accessed on 20 February 2014.

Baker, C. (2008) 'The power of learning through experience.' *Journal of Dementia Care 16*, 4, 27–29.

Baker, C. (2009) 'Introducing PEARL: rewarding good practice in dementia care.' *Journal of Dementia Care 17*, 4, 30–33.

Baker, C., and Edwards, P. (2002) 'The missing link: benchmarking person centred care.' *Journal of Dementia Care 10*, 6, 22–23.

Banerjee, S. (2009) *The Use of Antipsychotic Medication for People with Dementia: Time for Action*. London, UK: Department of Health.

Banerjee, S., Hellier, J., Romer, R., Dewey, M., Knapp, M., Ballard, C., Baldwin, R., Bentham, P., Fox, C., Holmes, C., Katona, C., Livingston, G., Lawton, C., McCrae, N., Moniz-Cook, E., Murray, J., Nurock, J., Orrell, M., O'Brien, J., Poppe, M., Thomas, A., Walwyn, R., Wilson, K., Burns, A. and Lindesay, J. (2013) 'Study of the use of antidepressants for depression in dementia: the HTA-SADD trial – a multicentre, randomised, double-blind, placebo-controlled trial of the clinical effectiveness and cost-effectiveness of sertraline and mirtazapine.' *Health Technology Assessment 17*, 7, 1–166.

Brooker, D. (1995) 'Looking at them, looking at me. A review of observational studies into the quality of institutional care for elderly people with dementia.' *Journal of Mental Health 4*, 2, 145–156.

Brooker, D. (2007) *Person-centred Dementia Care: Making Services Better*. London, UK: Jessica Kingsley Publishers.

Brooker, D. (2010) 'Quality: The Perspective of the Person with Dementia.' In M. Downs and B. Bowers (eds) *Excellence in Dementia Care: Research into Practice*. Maidenhead, UK: Open University, 476–492.

Brooker, D. and Surr, C. (2005) *Dementia Care Mapping: Principles and Practice*. Bradford, UK: University of Bradford.

Bryden, C. (2005) *Dancing with Dementia*. London, UK: Jessica Kingsley Publishers.

Cheston, R. and Byatt, C. (1999) 'Taped memories: a source of emotional security.' *Journal of Dementia Care 7*, 2, 28–29.

DH (Department of Health) (2001) *National Service Framework for Older People*. London, UK: DH.

DH (2009) *Living Well with Dementia: A National Dementia Strategy*. London, UK: DH.

DH (2010a) *The Essence of Care: Patient-focused Benchmarking for Healthcare Practitioners*. London: DH [originally published in 2001].

DH (2010b) *Equity and Excellence: Liberating the NHS (Nothing About Me)*. London, UK: DH.

DH (2012) *Transforming Care: A National Response to Winterbourne View Hospital, Department of Health Review: Final Report*. London, UK: DH.

DH (2013) *New Proposals to Ensure Care and Compassion in the NHS and in Social Care*. Available at www.gov.uk/government/news/new-proposals-to-ensure-care-and-compassion-in-the-nhs-and-in-social-care, accessed on 5 August 2013.

Ellis, J. (2002) 'Developing an interactive story for Margaret.' *Journal of Dementia Care 10*, 1, 16–17.

Feil, N. (1992) *Validation: the Feil Method. How to Help Disorientated Old-Old.* Jasper, OH: Edward Feil Productions.

Flynn, M. (2012) *Winterbourne View: A Serious Case Review.* Yate, UK: South Gloucestershire Safeguarding Adults Board. CPEA Ltd.

Francis, R. (QC) (2013) *Independent Inquiry into Care provided by Mid Staffordshire NHS Foundation Trust January 2005–March 2009.* Available at http://webarchive.nationalarchives.gov.uk/20130107105354/http://www.dh.gov.uk/prod_consum_dh/groups/dh_digitalassets/@dh/@en/@ps/documents/digitalasset/dh_113447.pdf, accessed on 3 October 2014.

FSHC (Four Seasons Health Care) (2013) *PEARL Dementia Care Report.* Available at www.fshc.co.uk/binary/CFh.pdf, accessed on 1 October 2013.

Gluzman, R., Meeker, H., Agarwal, P., Patel, S., Gluck, G., Espinoza, L., Ornstein, L., Soriano, T. and Katz, R.V. (2012) 'Oral health status and needs of home-bound elderly in an urban home-based primary care service.' *Special Care in Dentistry 33*, 5, 218–226.

Harwood, D. (2013) 'Good prescribing in dementia: a brief guide.' *The Journal of Dementia Care 21*, 4, 23–25.

Home & Medical (2014) *Dementia Care Living Aids.* Leeds. Available at www.homeandmedical.co.uk/research, accessed on 3 February 2014.

Horgas, A.L., McLennon, S.M. and Floetke, A.L. (2003) 'Pain management in persons with dementia.' *Alzheimer's Care Quarterly 4*, 4, 297–311.

Jacques, A. and Jackson, G.A. (2000) *Understanding Dementia* (3rd edition). London, UK: Harcourt Publishers.

James, I. and Stephenson, M. (2007) 'Behaviour that challenges us: the Newcastle Support Model.' *Journal of Dementia Care 15*, 5, 19–22.

Kitwood, T. (1997) *Dementia Reconsidered: The Person Comes First.* Buckingham, UK: Open University Press.

Kröpelin, T.F., Neyens, J.C.L., Halfens, R.J.G., Kempen, G.I.J.M. and Hamers, J.P.H. (2013) 'Fall determinants in older long-term care residents with dementia: a systematic review.' *International Psychogeriatrics 25*, 4, 549–563.

Martinez, C., Jones, R.W. and Rietbrock, S. (2013) 'Trends in the prevalence of antipsychotic drug use among patients with Alzheimer's disease and other dementias including those treated with anti-dementia drugs in the community in the UK: a cohort study.' *British Medical Journal Open 73*, 1, p.ii.

Mason, C. (1999) 'Guide to practice or 'load of rubbish': the influence of nursing care plans on nursing practice in five clinical areas in Northern Ireland.' *Journal of Advanced Nursing 29*, 2, 380–387.

Mitchell, G. and O'Donnell, H. (2013) 'The therapeutic use of doll therapy in dementia.' *British Journal of Nursing 22*, 6, 329–334.

Morrison, R.S. and Siu, A.L. (2000) 'A comparison of pain and its treatment in advanced dementia and cognitively intact patients with hip fracture.' *Journal of Pain and Symptom Management 19*, 4, 240–248.

Murphy, J., Oliver, T.M. and Cox, S. (2010) *Talking Mats Help Involve People with Dementia and the Carers in Decision Making*. York, UK: Joseph Rowntree Foundation.

Napp (2014) *Pain in People with Dementia: A Silent Tragedy*. London, UK: Napp Pharmaceuticals Limited.

Neubauer, D.N. (1999) 'Sleep problems in the elderly.' *American Family Physician 59*, 9, 2551–2558.

NICE (National Institute for Health and Care Excellence) (June 2013) *Falls: Assessment and Prevention of Falls in Older People*. Available at www.nice.org.uk/guidance/CG161, accessed on 14 February 2014.

NICE and SCIE (Social Care Institute for Excellence) (2011) *Dementia: Supporting People with Dementia and Their Carers in Health and Social Care*. NICE Clinical Guideline 42 2006-Revised 2011. London, UK: National Collaborating Centre for Mental Health.

Poston, B. (2009) 'An exercise in personal exploration: Maslow's hierarchy of needs.' *The Surgical Technologist*, August, 347–353.

Rolph, C.H. (1967) 'Cruelty in the Old People's Ward.' In B. Robb (ed.) *Sans Everything: A Case to Answer*. London, UK: Thomas Nelson & Sons.

Rubenstein, L.Z. (2006) 'Falls in older people: epidemiology, risk factors and strategies for prevention.' *Age Ageing 35*, 2, ii37–ii41.

Sabat, S. (1994) 'Excess disability and malignant social psychology – a case study of Alzheimer's disease.' *Journal of Community and Applied Social Psychology 4*, 157–166.

Sabat, S. (2010) 'A Bio-psycho-social Approach to Dementia.' In M. Downs and B. Bowers (eds) *Excellence in Dementia Care: Research into Practice*. Maidenhead, UK: Open University, 70–84.

Shah, S., Carey, I., Harris, T., Dewilde, S. and Cooke, D. (2011) 'Antipsychotic prescribing to older people living in care homes and the community in England and Wales.' *International Journal of Geriatric Psychiatry 26*, 4, 423–434.

Index

Page numbers in *italic* indicate figures.

Abbey Pain Scale 167–8, 174
'ABC' model of distress causation 166–7
abuse, of restraint 23–4, 157
acetylcholine receptors 122
adaptations 99
'adaptive behaviour' 111
admission/pre-admission process 45–6,
    82–3, 102, 174
    an imaginary experience with a person-
        centred approach 112–5
    an imaginary frightening experience
        107–10
agitation 121, 124–5
air cushions 78
air mattresses 78
analgesics *see* pain relief
anger 81, 125, 165–6
animals 141–2
anti-cholinergic drugs 122
anti-cholinesterase inhibitors 120
anti-depressants 52, 120, 122, 125–6, 178
anti-psychotic/sedating medication 19, 65,
    120–28
    and confusion 65, 123, 128
    evidence of physical harm 122–3
    historic background and current context
        119–21
    reduction with PEARL 16, 123–8, 174,
        183, 188–9
    sensory rooms used in preference to 'as
        required' medication 137–8
    side effects 120, 122–3
anti-spasmodic medication 122
anxiety 31, 124–5
    as a behavioural and psychological
        symptom 121
    and care plans 64
    and incontinence 170–2

and life story work 52–4
medication to reduce 52, 183 *see also* anti-
    depressants; SSRIs
and weight 64
audio recordings 55–6

Bacon, Sir Francis 162
Banerjee, S. 120, 122
Banks, Annette 185–6
bathing 23, 79–80
bathrooms 80, 133
    doors 130–1
bed, residents in 143–4
bedrooms 130–2
    tray service to 95–6, 186
behaviour analysis 166–70
    case study 170–2
    and distress reaction monitoring 166–9
behavioural and psychological symptoms
    (BPS) 120–5
best interest decisions 34, 37–45
    checklist *41–2*
    training 156
blame culture 63–4, 100
BPS (behavioural and psychological
    symptoms) 120–5
Braden Scale risk assessment 84
brain, acetylcholine receptors 122
Brooker, Dawn 16, 29, 92, 100, 153, 162
    VIPS framework approach *see* VIPS
        framework
Brown, Sarah 58–9
Bryden, Christine 28–9, 72, 111, 117, 194
    epigraphs 49, 105
Byatt, C. 56

Calveley, Pete 28
capacity assessments, Mental Capacity Act
    39–40

care plans 26, 61–72
    capturing points in 'general conversation'
        for 48
    documentation 151–2, 168–9
    evaluation of 65, 70
    labelling 152
    person-centred care planning training
        151–2
    person-centred examples 69–72
    to reduce distress 116
    resident/relative involvement in planning
        34, 36, 45–6, 66–72, 116 see also
        inclusion
    risk management plans 168–9
    shift from traditional 'medical model' to
        person-centred 61–72
    traditional (old culture) example 63–5
CD players 132–3
'challenging behaviour' 28, 85, 110–1,
        151, 166
    Newcastle Challenging Behaviour Service
        167
Cheston, R. 56
choice, resident see inclusion
citalopram 126
Clinical Practice Research Datalink 121
clothes see dressing
clothing protection, mealtime 101
cognitive impairment
    capacity assessment 39–40
    and care plans 64
    and consent 36
    and decision making 35–6, 39–45
    taking time over those with 75–6
colour
    of bedroom doors 130–1
    contrasts 95, 100, 133
    in corridors 134
    crockery colours 95, 99–100
    in lounge and dining areas 136
    in toilets 133
comfort 83–5
    pain relief see pain relief
    pressure relief 84–5
    and well-being 83–5
communication
    mealtime 96, 98–9
    non-verbal see non-verbal signs/
        communication
    reframing 116
confusion 95, 110, 121–2, 178
    disorientation 123, 176
    and sedative medication 65, 123, 128
consent 36

control 80, 82–3, 88, 100
    emotional 125
    see also disempowerment; independence
        facilitation
Cornell Depression Scale 167–8, 177–8
corridors 134, 184
crockery
    adapted 99
    coloured 95, 99–100
    plastic 101–2
cultural diets 102

daytime napping 87
DCM see Dementia Care Mapping™
decision making
    best interest see best interest decisions
    with cognitive impairment 35–6, 39–45
    covert medication administration scenario
        39–45
    every decision in everyday care 48
    historically denial of 35
    inclusion in 35–48
    with lack of verbal communication ability
        36
    and the Mental Capacity Act (2005) 34,
        36, 38–45
    and problematic answers 37–8
    with Talking Mats 40
Dementia 2013: A National Challenge 148
dementia care
    admission to a home see admission/pre-
        admission process
    benchmarks 26
    fundamental 73–88
    malignant social psychology in see
        malignant social psychology
    NICE guidelines for BPS 120
    person-centred see person-centred dementia
        care
    pharmacological see medication
    plans see care plans
    proactive see proactive care
    shift from old to new culture 61–72
Dementia Care Mapping™ (DCM) 25,
        32–3, 47, 121, 127, 154, 178–9
    evaluating the mealtime experience 103–4
    and sensory rooms 137–8
    training 154–5
Dementia Challenge, Prime Minister's 121
dementia prevalence 15, 119–20
denial 125
dentures 77, 80–1
depression 125–6, 167–8, 172
    Cornell Depression Scale 167–8, 177–8
    see also anti-depressants

Deprivation of Liberty Safeguards training 156
despair 125
digital frames 57
dignity 26
  in bathing 79–80
  at mealtimes 101–3
  in toilet care 78
dining rooms 136, 185–6
  furniture 95, 136
  size 96
disempowerment 25, 34, 65, 98–9, 102–3
disorientation 123, 176
disparagement 63, 99
distress 31, 33, 52–4
  'ABC' method of establishing cause of 166–7
  at being rushed 75, 110
  as BPS 121
  care plans to reduce 116
  framework and term of 'distressed reactions' 111–2, 151, 167–9
  frustration see frustration
  at mealtimes 64, 102–3
  monitoring of distress reaction 167–9
  non-pharmacological approaches to reducing distress/ distressed reactions 32, 48, 52–4, 80, 86, 105–16, 137–8
  non-verbal demonstrations of 81
  over bathing 80
  over preferences being ignored 68, 79, 102
  pharmacological treatment see anti-psychotic/sedating medication
  questions to help remember possible causes of 117
distress reaction monitoring 167–9
Do Not Attempt Resuscitation (DNAR) documentation 156
dogs 141–2
doll therapy 140–1, 186–7
doors
  bathroom 130–1
  bedroom 130–1
  'blended' locked doors 131, 134–5
  with glass panes 135
  toilet 130–1
dressing 79
  protective clothing 101
  resident choice in 82–3
drinking help 76–7
DVDs 56, 132

e-learning 149–50
eating see mealtimes
Ellis, Jim 55
Ellis, Margaret 55
embarrassment 74–5, 79, 170, 179
emotional responses to dementia 124–5
  emotional difficulties caused by treatment from others 149
  see also anger; anxiety; distress; embarrassment; frustration
empathy dolls 140–1
environment
  activities within the environment 140–5
  animals 141–2
  bathrooms see bathrooms
  bedrooms 130–2
  colour see colour
  corridors 134, 184
  developing a supportive environment 129–45
  doors see doors
  environmental cues 30
  external walls 138, 139
  garden areas 138–9
  household living 143
  lighting 134, 165
  lounge and dining areas 136
  mealtimes and the inclusive environment 94–6
  pictures see pictures
  reminiscence rooms 137, 137
  rest areas 135–6, 136
  room signage 94, 130
  sensory rooms 137–8
  supporting psychological needs 33–4
  toilets see toilets
Essence of Care 26–7
evaluation
  of care plans 65, 70
  of the mealtime experience 103–4
  through DCM see Dementia Care Mapping™
evidence-based observational techniques 123
  DCM see Dementia Care Mapping™
eye contact 98

falls, analysing and preventing 163–6, 176
fluoxetine 126
food/feeding help see mealtimes
foot care 81–2
Four Seasons Health Care
  Dementia Care Manual 28
  dining audit and mealtime experience 93

Four Seasons Health Care *cont.*
  foundations of person-centred care within
    27–9
  PEARL *see* PEARL (Positively Enriching
    And enhancing Residents' Lives)
    programme
  proactive care *see* proactive care
  staff training and support *see* staff training
    and support
Francis report 24
frosted glass 135
frustration 30–1, 65, 81, 83, 85, 124–5
  at being rushed 110
  at mealtimes 100, 102–3
  with reality orientation therapy 106
fundamental needs training 73

garden areas 138–9
General Practice Research Database 121
glass, frosted 135
guilt 74–5

Hechanova, Sister Yummy 186–7
Home from Home 148
household living 143
hydration 175–6
hypnotic medication 88, 165–6, 174, 183

inclusion
  in choice of bathing methods 79
  in choice of clothes 82–3
  in choice of meals 76, 96–8, 185
  in decision making 35–48
  mealtimes and the inclusive environment
    94–6
  and the Mental Capacity Act (2005) 36,
    38–45
  and natural person-centred care 34
  'Nothing About Me Without Me' phrase
    35
  of relatives *see* relative inclusion
  of whole staff team 157–8, 189–93
incontinence 116, 163
  and anxiety 170–2
independence facilitation 78, 98–101, 102,
    143, 163, 183

Jones, Sharon 29

Kitwood, Tom 25–6, 28, 63–4, 93, 101,
    148, 154
Kröpelin, T.F. 164

labelling 63, 85, 166, 167
  in care documentation 152
  see also 'challenging behaviour'
life story work 32, 49–60
  with audio recordings 55–6
  case studies 52–5, 59
  with digital frames 57
  with DVDs 56
  gathering information 55–60
  importance of life stories 49–52
  life story summaries 58–9
  and memorabilia 52–4
  with memory boxes 56–7, 132
  with music 56, 59–60
  as a navigation tool 60
  with photo albums 57
  for residents in bed 145
  and role continuity 50–2
  with story boards 58, 131
lifestyle, and role continuity 50–2
lighting 134, 165
lounges 136

malignant social psychology 25–6, 33–4,
    63, 112, 148–9
Martinez, C. 121, 126
Maslow's hierarchy of needs 74, *75*
Mason, C. 61
mealtimes 89–104, 183, 185–6
  adaptations for 99
  allowing time 77, 96, 98
  avoidance of medication administration
    94
  as busy periods in a care home 92
  chaotic 22
  colour contrasts to help item identification
    95
  communication at 96, 98–9
  cultural diets 102
  dignity at 101–3
  dining furniture 95
  dining room size 96
  distress at 64, 102–3
  evaluating the mealtime experience 103–4
  facilitating independence 98–102
  helping residents eat and drink well 76–7
  and the inclusive environment 94–6
  and mouth care 77
  music at 94
  noise levels 94
  nutritional intake 92–3, 175–6
  offering snacks to residents who wake in
    the night 87
  and PEARL 93–103

pleasant and unpleasant experiences of 90–94
portion size 77, 96, 98
residents' choice of food 76, 96–8, 185
table laying 95
timing of main meal 96
tray service 95–6, 186
Mebeverine 122
media, care industry hammering 23–4
medication
analgesic *see* pain relief
anti-cholinergic 122
anti-cholinesterase inhibitors 120
anti-depressant 52, 120, 122, 125–6, 178
anti-psychotic *see* anti-psychotic/sedating medication
anti-spasmodic 122
for anxiety reduction 52, 183 *see also* anti-depressants; SSRIs
avoidance of mealtime administration 94
baseline audits 172–3
covert administration of 39–45
and falls 165–6
hypnotic 88, 165–6, 174, 183
Parkinson's treatments 122
psychotropic 165–6
'sedating' *see* anti-psychotic/sedating medication
and weight loss 65
memorabilia 52–4, 131, 142
memory boxes 56–7, 132
Mental Capacity Act (2005) 34, 36, 38–45, 156
capacity assessment 39–40
training 156
menu choice 76, 96–8, 185
mood analysis 176–9
mouth care 77, 80–1
music 56, 59–60
at mealtimes 94

Napp Pharmaceuticals Limited 124
napping, daytime 87
National Dementia Strategy 30, 121, 165
National Health Service and Community Care Act (1990) 24
National Service Framework for Older People 26
Newcastle Challenging Behaviour Service 167
NICE (National Institute for Health and Care Excellence) 120, 126
non-verbal signs/communication 32–3, 75, 78, 83, 85, 88, 99

cues 43
eye contact 98
prompts 99
room signage 94, 130
nutritional intake 92–3, 175–6
see also mealtimes
observation 32, 48, 123, 127
to evaluate mealtime experience 103–4
evidence-based techniques 123 *see also* Dementia Care Mapping™ (DCM)
opiate analgesics 122
Optimising Treatment and Care for People with Behavioural and Psychological Symptoms of Dementia 126
oral health 77, 80–1
Oxybutynin 122

pain
Abbey Pain Scale 167–8, 174
analysing 172–4
dental 80–1
management training 156
as a possible cause of distress 167–8
recognising when a resident is in pain 32, 48, 81
unmanaged/poorly managed 124
pain relief 52–3, 78, 84, 124, 166, 173–4
ineffective 173
opiate analgesics 122
PEARL (Positively Enriching And enhancing Residents' Lives) programme 15–6, 87–8
anti-psychotic medication reduction with 16, 123–8, 174, 183, 188–9
distress reduction with 107–17
introductory extracts of a fictional journey 107–10, 112–5
launch of 29
and mealtimes 93–103
outcome successes for relatives 187–9
outcome successes for residents 182–7
outcome successes for staff 189–93
outcome successes for whole organisation 193–4
proactive care *see* proactive care
reports 99
staff training and support *see* staff training and support
weight gain with 16, 77, 104, 183
well-being increased with 16
person-centred dementia care 21–34
DCM *see* Dementia Care Mapping™
Dementia Care Manual 28
development from end of the 1990s 25–7

person-centred dementia care *cont.*
  and dignity *see* dignity
  dressing *see* dressing
  early years of 22–3
  eating and drinking help *see* mealtimes
  embedding the ethos of 16
  enabling good sleep 85–8
  and the environment *see* environment
  evaluation *see* evaluation
  facilitating independence 78, 98–102,
      143, 163, 183
  foot care 81–2
  foundations within Four Seasons Health
      Care 27–9
  fundamental care 73–88
  imaginary admission experience with a
      person-centred approach 112–5
  inclusion *see* inclusion
  and life stories *see* life story work
  and media hammering of care industry
      23–4
  medication *see* medication
  mouth care 77, 80–1
  naturalness of 34
  non-verbal communication in *see* non-
      verbal signs/communication
  origins 24–5
  plans *see* care plans
  proactive *see* proactive care
  resident comfort *see* comfort
  respect in *see* respecting residents
  role continuity activities 50–2
  skin care *see* skin care
  staff support *see* staff training and support
  time to care *see* time to care
  tools *see* tools for dementia care
  training *see* staff training and support
  validation of care homes 181–2
  VIPS framework *see* VIPS framework
  washing 23, 79–80
personal hygiene 78–82
  see also toilet care
photo albums 57
pictures 48, 56
  on bedroom doors 131
  in corridors 134
  digital frames 57
  on external walls 138, *139*
  photo albums 57
  in room signage 130
planters 139, *139*
plastic crockery 101–2
Poston, B. 74
pressure relief 84–5

pressure sores 22, 73, 78
Prime Minister's Dementia Challenge 121
proactive care 33, 64, 112, 161–79
  analysing behaviour *see* behaviour analysis
  analysing/preventing falls 163–6, 176
  analysing mood 176–9
  analysing pain 172–4
  analysing weight loss 175–6
  with DCM *see* Dementia Care Mapping™
  in oral health 81
  training and skills for analysing
      information 162
Procyclidine 122
prompts 99
protective clothing 101
psychotropic medication 165–6

quality of life 88, 92, 154, 163, 169, 176–9
  proactive fostering of *see* proactive care
  see also well-being

reading to residents 145
reality orientation therapy 106
relative inclusion 34, 36, 45–6, 66–8, 116,
      123, 171–2, 186
  and outcome successes for relatives 187–9
relaxation DVDs 132
reminiscence rooms 137, *137*
repositioning regimes 78
resident choice *see* inclusion
resident experience training 28, 112, 153,
      185
resident perspective 32–3, 88
  training to gain *see* resident experience
      training
respecting residents 74–5
  with dignity *see* dignity
  helping them be comfortable 83–5
  by inclusion *see* inclusion
  by person-centred care *see* person-centred
      dementia care
  without putting them at risk 116 *see also*
      risk assessment; risk management
      care plans
rest areas 135–6, *136*
restraint 23–4, 156–7
  training requests by regulators 156
risk assessment 84, 100, 141, 164
risk management care plans 168–9
risk taking 100
  mobility and the risk of falling 163–6
risperidone 127
role continuity activities 50–2

Rolph, C.H. 22
room signage 94, 130
routines 22–3
    awareness of resident's preferred routines
        79, 115
    bathing 22, 79–80
    mealtime 22
    night time 23
    person-centred 31–2
    sleep patterns 86
    toilet 23, 78
Rubenstein, L.Z. 163–4
rummage boxes 142

Sabat, S. 92, 149
sadness 125
sedation/sedatives see anti-psychotic/sedating
    medication
Selective Serotonin Reuptake Inhibitors
    (SSRIs) 126
self-actualisation (Maslow) 74
self-esteem 51, 80
sensory rooms 137–8
sensory trays 144, 145
sertraline 126
signage, room 94, 130
simulated presence therapy 55–6
skin care 77–8
    of the feet 81–2
sleep 85–8
    daytime napping 87
    disturbed 87, 172
snack boxes 101
SSRIs (Selective Serotonin Reuptake
    Inhibitors) 126
staff successes 189–93
staff training and support 147–60
    and accreditation 159
    for analysing information 162
    bespoke training 156–7
    DCM training 154–5
    development programmes 155–6
    e-learning 149–50
    fundamental needs training 73
    general nurse training covering of
        dementia care 148
    inclusion of whole staff team 157–8
    person-centred care planning 151–2
    person-centred care training 150–1
    resident experience training 28, 112,
        153, 185
    rewards of 159–60
    supervision and support meetings 157–8
    with VIPS framework 158

staff turnover 189
stained glass 135
story boards 58, 131
support for staff see staff training and support

table laying 95
Talking Mats 40
tearfulness 71, 121, 125
time to care 75–6
    at mealtimes 77, 96, 98
toenails 81
toilet care 23, 78
toilets
    decor 133
    doors 130–1
tools for dementia care
    benchmarking 26
    depression and well-being tools for mood
        analysis 167–8, 176–9
    distress reaction monitoring 166–9
    navigational 60 see also life story work
    observational see Cornell Depression
        Scale; Dementia Care Mapping™
        (DCM); distress reaction monitoring;
        observation; vision, seeing the needs
        of a patient
    for pain management see Abbey Pain Scale;
        pain relief
    risk assessment tools 84
    therapies see doll therapy; reality
        orientation therapy; simulated
        presence therapy; validation therapy
training see staff training and support
tray service 95–6, 186
tricyclic anti-depressants 122

unfamiliarity 87, 123

validation of care homes 181–2
validation therapy 106–7
valuing people 30–1
VIPS framework 16, 29–34, 149
    individualised approaches (I) 31–2
    perspective of the resident (P) 32–3
    social environment that supports
        psychological needs (S) 33–4
    staff support concerning 158
    valuing people (V) 30–1
vision, seeing the needs of a patient 48
    see also observation
visual media 56
vitamins 176
vulnerability 22, 80–1

washing 23, 79–80
Waterlow score 84
weight
    and anxiety 64
    increased with PEARL 16, 77, 104, 183
    loss 65, 77, 102, 175–6
    and medication 65
    monitoring 65
    proactive analysis of weight loss 175–6
well-being
    care plans for *see* care plans
    and comfort 83–5
    increased with PEARL 16
    and life story work 32, 54–5
    and mood analysis 176–9
    and pain management 173 *see also* pain
        relief
    and personal preferences 82–3
    proactive fostering of *see* proactive care
    and quality of life 88, 92, 154, 163, 169,
        176–9
    and role continuity 50–1
    tools 176–9
    and weight loss 175–6
    Well-being Profiling Tool 167–8, 177–8
Winterbourne View abuse scandal 23–4, 157
work stations 143